THE BEST:
A Life Manifesto

A Practical Guide to Making Your Life Count

By: GP Hintz

© 2011

Copyright © 2011 GP Hintz

All rights reserved.

ISBN: 0615556248
ISBN-13: 978-0615556246

THE BEST: A Life Manifesto

A GP Enterprise Book
Published by GP Enterprise
Copyright © 2011 by GP Hintz

All rights reserved. No part of this publication may be reproduced, stored in a retrieval system or transmitted in any form or by any means – electronic, mechanical, photocopying, recording, or otherwise – without written permission.

THE BEST: a life manifesto / GP Hintz
ISBN: 0615556248
ISBN-13: 978-0615556246

Dedicated to those individuals who are refusing to accept a mediocre life or a mundane existence… to those who have a fire in their hearts and a belief in their soul that they are created for something more…

This book is for you!

TABLE OF CONTENTS

1	The Beginning	2
2	The Feet: *Living a Life of Purpose*	9
3	The Sphincter: *Getting the Crap out of Your Life*	27
4	The Hands: *The Stuff of Life*	51
5	The Lungs: *The Breath of Life*	73
6	The Mouth: *The Lingo of Life*	92
7	The Brain: *Mental Development*	107
8	The Eyes: *A Window to the Soul*	121
9	The Arm Pit: *Controlling the Negative Odors of Life*	138
10	The Brawn: *Pump You Up!*	151
11	The Ears: *Listening for Life*	169
12	The Soul: *Spiritual Awakening*	186
13	Epilogue: *The End is Really the Beginning*	205
	Endnotes	208

ACKNOWLEDGMENTS

As I look over my life, the number of people who have believed in me can't be counted. I seek here not to make an exhaustive list, but simply to list a few as a personal thank you from me to you.

To my beautiful wife Tara... I wouldn't be half the man I am without your love and support. Thank you.

To my dad... you have proved to be a foundation layer in my life and I owe my life to your investments. Thank you.

To my mom... you made me into the man I am. May my life make you proud. Thank you.

To my wonderful children... you have taught me how to smile and cause my days to be filled with a greater joy. Thank you.

To Saemus and Roger... you are as different as can be, but have both proved to be brothers to me. Thank you.

To the wonderful faith community at THE PLACE... you have taught me love, passion and purpose like no other. Thank you.

To the countless people who never lost hope in me... this book is as much yours as it is mine. Thank you.

To all my friends and family... I love you guys so much! You inspire me and make me a better man. Thank you.

Most of all, I want to thank God... You have provided me with the faith and tenacity to hold on and never give up. Thank you.

"For I know the plans I have for you...plans to prosper you and not to harm you. Plans to give you a hope and a future."
Jeremiah 29:11

1

The Beginning

"Every new beginning comes
from some other beginning's end."

—Seneca *(Roman philosopher—mid-1ˢᵗ century AD)*

I never imagined that it would happen the way it did…700 miles from home in a rented out beach house. I knew that the day would eventually come; but not that day or in that way. I could have seen it happening when she was diagnosed with cancer or after her first major heart attack, but not on the first day of a major family vacation. This place was supposed to be about victory and overcoming and fun. Instead, it smelled of death and provided memories which made it hard to sleep at night.

We loaded into a van jam-packed from front to back. There were bags filled with games for the kids and coolers packed to capacity with food and swim trunks and boogie boards and suitcases and diapers. We crammed into our respective seats and received a comfort that is only provided by family and a peace which comes only from the presence of those you love.

The drive went faster than expected—too quick in light of the circumstances. We traveled from Northeast Ohio to Cape Hatteras, North Carolina. A trip filled with flat lands then mountains then flat lands then sea. We went nonstop, taking turns at the wheel and sharing the duty of driving. I preferred the night and saw us through the moon-filled moments while

Mom snored in the back and I passed the time talking politics with Dad. The kids were fast asleep, bobbing to the motion of the bumps, and my wife's eyes were closed and silent.

Sunset arrived as we drove into the seaside town. Surfboards and seascape filled the driver's side window and I vividly remembered this place, being here twice in the past. The National Seashore spanned to both horizons and the sand dune prohibited me from seeing the endless rhythm of the ocean. I longed for its breath to breathe on me, feeling its mist on my face. I knew that the upcoming week would provide many opportunities for its touch, so I sat and patiently waited.

We picked up the key to our rented out beach house and rushed to the stilted bungalow. Choosing our bedrooms, we quickly unloaded the van, leaving our seaside escape filled with boxes and bags which would bring us comfort in the days to come. Our hunger led us to a local dive down the street.

The sun was setting and the air was warm on our skin as we pulled into the restaurant parking lot. The kids exited the car with a skip in their step, happy to be freed from its grasp. My mom played with her grandsons on the ramp of the restaurant—chasing them up, then running down backward in front of them, making sure that they didn't fall. We sat and drank and ate and laughed, breathing deep the joy of the moment. Mom loved to laugh and her smile was contagious.

We ended up back at our rented house after the sun had set, but my deep desire for the rhythm of the waves could no longer be held back—I had to see the ocean. Asking my parents, they agreed and we all headed off to the beach. Having to walk down a few streets and a couple of football fields' worth of sand, the hike took a little bit longer than I had expected, but was well worth it when we hit the apex of the dune and tasted the salt air on our tongues. I ran ahead with the kids, eager for them to witness the power and rage of the ocean at night. My parents were lagging behind; sharing in a romantic moment—at least that is what I thought.

We spent some time on the beach and then headed back to the house. I made my mom a nightcap and indulged in one myself. My wife was prodding her to enter the Jacuzzi—a must have on a vacation—and she finally gave in; always up for a good time. I snuck away, beneath the house, to partake in a cigarette I had taken from my mom's pack. I was in my mid twenties and still stealing cigarettes from my mom's never ending pack. I'm not sure if it was that I really wanted to smoke or if I was in the mood to do something 'bad'. Either way, I partook.

I hadn't taken three puffs when I heard the incessant screaming from the house. At first, I assumed that my mom and wife were just having fun teasing each other on who would throw who into the Jacuzzi. As the screams went to shrieks, I threw my cigarette on the ground and ran around the house. I saw my dad dragging my mom's limp body through the doorframe and I jumped to help him; grabbing her legs to put her on the couch. In a flash, my mind traveled back to the days when I worked as an EMT driving an ambulance. I didn't know any of those people, though; I was not fruit of their womb.

Her breath was shallow and sporadic and I couldn't feel her heartbeat. I didn't know what to do. My dad began yelling to call 911. My wife dialed the number with shaky fingers and I did the only thing I knew how to do—I started CPR.

I couldn't remember if it was three pumps and one breath or five pumps and two breaths. I guess it didn't matter anyway. **I pumped and breathed and pumped and breathed and cried in my heart—in a place where no one could see. The sirens rang far away and I continued. Three pumps. One breath. Four Pumps. Two breaths. Two Pumps. "Hurry up! Hurry up!"**

I couldn't see my dad, but I knew that he was only two breaths away and I could feel his presence and the palm of his hand pressed hard against his teeth—biting against reality. Before me, under my 'pumps' existed the woman that he had loved since she was fifteen years old. The lips that I pressed hard against were those that had been kissed in a church in Hawaii on their wedding day and on a white sand beach on their wedding night. She had, in many ways, been his reason for existence and now she lay limp beneath my fingers.

The police men were followed by the firefighters who were followed by the EMTs who were followed by the paramedics who were followed by the longest thirty minutes of my life. With a defibrillator providing shocks of voltage throughout her body and the sound of my wife's tears in the next room and the gawking eyes of North Carolinians looking at my mom's exposed body, I had no thought and no emotion. I resembled a shell of a man—one who existed but didn't feel, one with bones but no soul.

They loaded her in the ambulance and I drove my dad 90 miles per hour in a van that had much better pickup than it did six hours before. The hospital was a lifetime away and my dad's tears and words exposed his hopelessness. "What am I going to do if I lose her? I can't lose her. I can't. She's everything to me.

She's everything…" His words drifted off then came back to the beginning and repeated themselves. What more was there to say?

The hospital looked like an abandoned school and a doctor who looked like he had just woken up met my mom at the door. At that moment I wished that I hadn't worked in an emergency room for seven years, because I could tell by the faces of the paramedics that there was no beating heart or breathing patient. The doctor's job was not to save a life tonight, but explain its loss to a hurting husband and an absent son. We sat and waited for the inevitable: the news that my mom had died of a massive heart attack at the age of 54.

> **"People fear death even more than pain. It's strange that they fear death. Life hurts a lot more than death. At the point of death, pain is over. Yeah, I guess it is a friend."**
>
> —**Jim Morrison** *(lead singer of "The Doors")*

The news came quick and was swallowed hard—by both my dad and I. A priest was called, but never showed up. The ambulance driver sat behind a pale desk and filled out his paperwork—afraid to look into the whites of our eyes. I knew that feeling: doing a job that affected people who you wished didn't exist. I knew that feeling well.

This moment changed me forever. It brought a greater definition to who am I and who I am to become. One of the darkest moments of my life proved to bring the greatest light. I chose to embrace my life differently after that day and I chose to make my life count. I chose to begin to live according to a popular quote, "Live your life to the fullest" which also rests on the face of my mom's headstone.

This book is a testament to that moment and to my mom and to the reality that there is a deep well of potential and opportunity that is resting just below the surface of our lives. For many, this well lies untapped, but the goal of this work is to empower us to take the bucket of potential and plunge it deep into those cool, refreshing waters. By doing this, you will begin to create a crystal-clear path to the future that you desire and the destiny that you were created to fulfill.

This is not just a book… this is a Manifesto. In the same way that there have been works written that have painted the plans of everyone from the Communists in the 'Communist Manifesto' to the Humanists in the 'Humanist Manifesto', I believe that your life is worth having a manifesto. Your life is worth having a plan and a direction and a destination. Your life is worth putting forth the thoughts and attention that others have put forth for organizations or societal revolutions. Many of us are in desperate need of a life revolution and this work is designed to do exactly that: bring a personal revolution that will change your life forever.

This is not a passive expression of thoughts and ideas, but a proactive tool that is going to become your personal manifesto. You will be able to take from it as much as you are willing to put into it. If you are only looking for static ideas to place in your mind for a few days and then on the bookshelf for the next twenty years, you will be thoroughly disappointed. If, however, you are looking for an interactive guide to bring the quality of your existence up for the remainder of your life, you have chosen the right book!

The key to the level of change that you will experience from this work will be directly linked to your participation. In each chapter you will be asked to become involved with your life. You will have to think about where you currently are and where you want to end up. You will have to answer some tough questions and uncover some things that may have been buried for a long time. The payoff, however, will be amazing. When all is said and done you will have a living document that you can refer back to and update and change as the path of your life unfolds before you.

So, without any further commentary, I want you to dive in and get ready, because you are now beginning a journey that will change everything. I hope you are ready to begin living THE BEST life ever! Because you are now beginning a journey that is sure to lead you there...

2

The Feet: Living a Life of Purpose

> "My conviction that 'the work is His' —is more than reality. —I have never doubted. It hurts me when the people call me foundress because I know for certain He asked—'Will you do this for me?' Everything was His—I had only to surrender myself to His plan—to His will. — Today, His work has grown because it is He, not I, that do it through me. Of this I am convinced—that I would give my life gladly to prove it…"
>
> —Mother Teresa *(20th century Missionary to India)*

I can think of no other person who exudes the picture of living a life of purpose than Mother Teresa. Here is a woman who, at the great stature of four foot ten, inspired an entire world and was able to transcend sex and culture and every barrier known to man. Catholics lift her up as a Saint while Agnostics praise her for her humanitarianism. Countless people have entered into a life of sacrifice because of her example, but it didn't start out that way.

Imagine a woman born at the turn of the 20th century in the country of Macedonia with a name like Agnes Gonxha Bojaxhiu. She felt a strong call from God at the age of twelve and joined a convent at the age of eighteen. After a few months she found herself in the country of India serving at a school and teaching for over seventeen years. Then, after receiving permission to leave the school and start working among the poorest of the poor in India, she set out on a journey of servitude. In 1950 she started the Missionaries of Charity which is an organization still working tirelessly throughout the world to serve those in extreme poverty.

I always look at Mother Teresa as someone who had a firm understanding of her purpose. I see a woman who never seemed to waver from what she believed to be her *calling* and I have always greatly admired her for that. It is not that everything always went perfect for her—because it didn't. But even when things didn't go just the way that she desired, she stayed the course and was able to accomplish amazing things with her life.

"We can do no great things. Only small things with great love"

—**Mother Teresa** *(founder of the Missionaries of Charity)*

I have desired this same clear vision and strong tenacity about the life that I am called to live and, over the years, I have met many others who long for this too. *How are we able to get to the place where we are living a life of purpose? How can we assure that we are truly making a difference with our life?*

The first step to living a life of fulfillment is to have a clear understanding of one word—'purpose'. We need to understand what this word means and we need to build from this place of understanding. And at the very core of this word *purpose* is its meaning... "an aim or an intention". It is also defined as "an object to be reached, a target, or a goal". So, in order to live a life of purpose, we need to know the direction where we want to see ourselves moving. We need to have a clear vision of the target.

There are so many of us who are simply drifting in the currents of life. We are moving, but we are not directing our lives. It is simply the currents of culture or family or career or relationships. We are floating—or existing—but there is no real purpose behind that existence except to take up space. We don't even really think too much about the life that we are living until we face some extreme travesty or traumatic event. We aren't living a life of *purpose*, but living a life of *existence* from day to day.

Begin to ask yourself, what is the goal of my life? What do I want to be known for? There are many who are reaching for selfish goals, but those goals are flawed and will never bring about the satisfaction that they think they will. For example, I meet many people who believe that the ultimate goal for life has a dollar sign in front of it. However, this dollar sign can never be the 'end all' of life because this simply initiates the chase of the proverbial carrot. When do you know you're there? When do you have *enough*? You keep striving after money and this insatiable hunger in your heart can never be satisfied.

And even if you find yourself able to ascertain money, your job now becomes to protect it. If you are emotionally tied to this money, how are you going to react when it disappears? I promise you, it will eventually all disappear. You could lose it overnight as many did in the recent stock market drop of 2008—2009. The only thing you heard on the news was how the sky was falling and for many it was literally the end of their lives because everything that they had trusted in was gone. The carrot had been eaten and there was no longer a reason for their existence.

Others believe that their purpose resides in stuff. If they can just get that next great thing then their life will have a greater depth of meaning. The next car or boat or vacation or TV or house drives them to get up and 'make the donuts' each day, but when we finally get these things, they often become a let down and don't provide us with the satisfaction that we thought they would.

I will never forget the day that I bought my first—and last—Cadillac. It wasn't just any Cadillac, but it was a sporty model with leather seats, a moon roof and power everything. It was fast and made me feel like a 'somebody'. It is amazing what that little Cadillac symbol can do to a person's sense of self worth. I should have done a little better research though, because the Cadillac that I bought was a Cadillac Catera.

This sporty model began being offered to the public in 1999 and had prided itself in all of the bells and whistles, but the shine quickly began to fade with the emergence of problems like initial tire wear issues, faulty oil coolers, and engine failures due to timing belt tensioner failures. I will never forget the problems that began to consume my car... and my life. I had found that my dream car had become my lemon and was sucking away my life both emotionally and financially. This car became the weight carrying me under the sea of life. **This car taught me that stuff never satisfies.**

Others may believe that the purpose of life lies within them. They have the thought that "If I could just look like this or that" or "If I could just get this degree or that degree" or "If I could just get this perfect job in this perfect place". Unfortunately however, when we get these *external* things, the glitter goes away and the shine begins to dull and we're left holding a *product* that is never as good as the *advertisement*. None of these things that we looked at are inherently evil in and of themselves, but if they become the entirety of our lives, then they are sure to leave us lacking and empty.

We need to discover how to tap into a deeper and richer place when it comes to purpose. We have to dig deep into the bowels of our souls and try to discover what really gets us excited about life. You can find this out by asking yourself some simple questions. Let's look at a few of these now. I want you to grab a pen, pencil or computer and literally answer these questions right here and right now:

What do you like to talk about with friends?

_____
_____
_____
_____
_____
_____
_____

What gets you excited when you think about it?

_____
_____
_____
_____
_____
_____
_____

What keeps you up at night thinking, processing and planning?

_____
_____
_____
_____
_____
_____
_____

If you didn't have to work, what would you fill your days with?

_____
_____
_____
_____
_____
_____
_____

What do you like to teach other people?

_____
_____
_____
_____
_____
_____

I hope that as you were answering these questions that you were able to begin to see a theme starting to work its way to the surface. A lot of times it may be something like a passion for music… other times it could be reading or writing… or possibly traveling or animals… or even serving others or business. None of these answers are better than the others because they reflect you and who you are and what you love. In order to discover **purpose** we need to discover **passion**. Purpose always follows passion so it's imperative that we start from a place of passion.

"Nothing great in the world has ever been accomplished without passion."

—Christian Friedrich Hebbel
(A 19th century German poet and dramatist)

Now, I am going to ask you to do one of the hardest things that you have ever been asked to do. **I want you to *forget about the money*.** Even if your passion was business or entrepreneurship or finances in general, I need you to simply forget about the cash… the greenbacks… the bucks. When money is our motivator, it is too easy to become discouraged and give up. Set cash to the side and begin to focus on your passion.

If money wasn't an issue, what would you do? Now that you've looked at some things that get your juices flowing, what would you do? Pina Coladas and hammocks on the beach are probably really fun for the first six months or so, but eventually it gets old. What would you do with your time if you didn't **have** to do anything with it? How would you invest your days… your nights… your early mornings? What would you reach for? What would you strive towards? What would your life look like?

Take some time and answer these next few questions:

Working with the passion that we just uncovered, what would you like to see yourself doing with this passion in the next time periods:

1 month:

_____
_____
_____
_____
_____
_____
_____
_____
_____

6 months:

_____
_____

THE BEST: A Life Manifesto

_____
_____
_____
_____
_____
_____
_____
_____

1 year:

_____
_____
_____
_____
_____
_____
_____
_____
_____
_____

5 years:

_____
_____
_____
_____
_____
_____
_____
_____
_____
_____

30 years:

_____
_____
_____
_____
_____
_____
_____
_____
_____
_____

This exercise may have been very difficult for you for one or more reasons. Maybe you had no problem with the one month goal, but when it came down to 5–30 years, it was more difficult. What could this passion turn into in thirty years? Maybe your mind has difficulty seeing that far in the future. Or, on the other hand, maybe some of you had a crystal clear idea of what it looks like in 30 years, but had no idea what to write in the one month to one year category. For you, you know where you want to be but you have absolutely no idea on how to get there. **Either way, you are in a great place to begin because now you are beginning to understand what your passion is.**

This is the moment for you to get busy about creating the life that you desire. Oftentimes you will hear this concept of "reaching out and going for it" in faiths from the west to the east. I am reminded of a story from the New Testament of the Bible with Jesus who is walking on the water. One of his disciples, Peter, looks to him and says: *"If it's you, tell me to come to you on the water."* He does and Peter walks on water. Or, I also think of the words of Lao-Tzu who is the father of Taoism who said, *"The journey of 1000 miles begins with a single step."* This is the place where you are today. You are about to walk on water and go on a journey. Your personal life journey is going to begin with your leg going over the side of the boat and starting to walk those 1000 miles.

These first steps are going to begin with action. Any major, lasting change in your life needs to be attributed to your action. You have to enter the fight and be busy about bringing about the change that needs to happen in your life. You have the heard the proverb, *"The road to hell is paved with good intentions."* The *hell* of your life is simply staying the same or treading the water or maintaining the status quo that you have been sustaining for all this time. You want a change in your life; now you have to get busy bringing about that change that you want to see. It is truly the difference between you *wanting* something to happen and *ensuring* something to happen. **You** are the only guarantee for the life that you long for.

Gandhi said, *"Become the change that you want to see in the world."* I would take that to a microcosmic level and say: *"Become the change that you want to see in your life."* It is only when we do this that we are going to be able to truly change the world.

THE GREATER GOOD

Personally, this self discovery has taken me many different places throughout the world and to many dark corners of my own soul. I have traveled this road many times and its cement has led me to places of darkness and despair. However, its path has also allowed me to tap into true love and understanding that has only come from a greater understanding of myself and the purpose for my existence… and it is nothing like I ever expected.

One journey took place in the summer of 1999 when my wife and I had signed up to go overseas and work in the city of Rio de Janeiro, Brazil. My only encounters with this city had been in tourist books and travel videos which highlighted the colorful Carnivale and beautiful beaches. Needless to say, I couldn't wait to 'serve' this poor, misguided city. *(Shhhhh. I was in it for the beaches ;-)*

I'll never forget landing in this country and realizing that everything that I had read and saw in the videos was absolutely true. Brazil was the most beautiful place that I had ever been. The waves were lapping the white sand beaches as the palm trees glided back and forth in the breeze. People walked on the sidewalks with sun kissed bodies and everyone seemed to be smiling. We made it to our hotel and nestled in for the night. I opened my window and let the sweet, salty air pour into my room. This was truly the life.

The next day I discovered that the work that we were to be doing wasn't going to be with the surfers across from the hotel, but that we were traveling into an area of the city known as a 'favela'. This was the first time that I had ever heard this term used, and because it was a Portuguese word that I had no reference for, I quickly dismissed it and remained excited for what the day would hold.

We drove less than an hour to the favela where we were to be serving. I wasn't ready for what I saw from my bus window. People were everywhere and children were dirty and barely clothed. Dogs roamed the streets, dirty and mangy, searching for food and fearful of man. The houses... if that is what you would call them... were made of plywood or cardboard or cinder blocks. Really, they were made with whatever could be found. Garbage boxing in families. The bus parked.

I exited the bus and waited for instructions, moving my wallet from my back pocket to the front as I had been warned to do in my travel videos. I touched my chest and felt my passport resting securely in my security bag which hung around my neck. My eyes shifted quickly from the left to the right, striving to take it all in without making eye contact with anyone.

My group began to move and I was relieved. I felt safer moving in the group. I could travel to the center like a sickly calf in the midst of the herd. There was a safety in numbers and it made me breathe easier. We met our contact from inside the favela that wore a large toothed smile and made me feel secure. I touched my front pocket. I was safe.

We were told that we were going to be hosting a health clinic for the favela and that most of the families in these slums had never seen a doctor. The children never had vaccinations and disease ran rampant through these families. Our job was simple, travel with a translator and let them all know that we were opening a clinic for them the next day. It seemed effortless. I attached myself to my group and began my trek into the favela.

I had never experienced poverty like this. There was a trench that ran down the middle of the street. It stunk and children hopped back and forth over it like a gazelle dashing through a field. I asked the translator what it was. He replied kindly, *"Oh sir... that is the sewage. It runs like a river."* I looked again at the kids playing by puddles of piss and my heart sank.

We came to the dwelling of a woman whose two children who had just returned from work. They were probably aged six and eight and sold Chiclet gum at a stoplight on the main highway. Cars would stop at the light and they would walk down next to the cars selling pieces of gum to the people for pennies. This gum money was their only income and was how they would eat each day. Having just sold out, they were now home for more pieces to peddle.

She let us in the home and her *home*, if you can call it that, was smaller than my walk in closet. A family of three living in my walk in closet. The shower was behind the house in the open—basically a hose hung from a hook. There was only one small bed and a hot plate for food. I remember looking at this 'home' and thinking to myself, 'How can people live like this?'

But what I remember more than anything wasn't the size of the house, but the size of the smile on this woman and her two children. They were happy. They loved each other and they were living their lives together. I remember wanting to grab them and shake them and tell them, *"Quit smiling! You're not supposed to be happy. You don't have anything. You are supposed to be sad and angry about this. What is wrong with you?"* But they simply smiled, offered us some food (which we didn't take) and thanked us profusely for bringing the health clinic to their favela. They told us that they would be there the next day. We left that home and I was never the same again.

"Things do not change; we change."

—**Henry David Thoreau** *(a 19th century American poet, author and abolitionist)*

That memory singed itself to the lower lobe of my brain and I couldn't forget their smiles and the love that I sensed from their presence. **I was missing something.** I thought that the goal of life was to get promotions and a bigger house and a shinier car. I had been pursuing all of these things, yet could never find the smile that this impoverished family had. I knew that I wanted the smile more than the stuff. I just felt like the only way that I could get that smile was through the stuff. I realized how wrong I was to pursue a smile in a pile of things. The smile that I longed had been lying within my reach for all this time, but I was simply looking in the wrong place for it.

This smile that expressed peace and love and joy and contentment… this smile that had been my longing for many years had come to me. **In the midst of piss and Chiclet gum, it came to me. In the midst of squalor and filth, it came to me. I had traveled to another part of the globe to help change people and realized that the one that changed the most was I.**

I remained in Brazil for another week and a half and found my smile in the heart of the favelas. We served the people and their medical needs. There were lines awaiting medical attention over 2 city blocks long. We saw mothers and babies and children. We sang songs with them and played in the streets. We hugged people. We fed people. We loved people. And I found my smile there.

You see, when we talk about purpose, true joy comes from a place of service to others. When we decide in our hearts that we want to pour our lives out for the needs of others, there is a deep sense of peace that pours over us. The ultimate sacrifice on the path of discovering your true purpose is simply **self**. We must learn to sacrifice **self** to find our **self**. It is truly a paradigm shift of epic proportions.

There is a deep, lasting satisfaction from serving the needs of others. There is a serenity that is tapped into the DNA of service. Other people have to be tied in with our purpose or we find ourselves creating a lonely existence. I love how Stephen Covey put it in his famous work, *The Seven Habits of Highly Effective People* as he discusses the importance of a win/win relationship:

"Win/Win is a frame of mind and heart that constantly seeks mutual benefit in all human interactions." [2]

—**Stephen Covey** *(a 20th century American author)*

We will begin to find blessing and abundance poured out into our lives when we simply take the eyes off of only ourselves and look for ways to use our passions to serve others. How can my music inspire a generation? How can my investment strategies benefit third world poverty? How can this idea I have improve the lives of more people than just my immediate family and I? Expand your thoughts and ideas to include more than just you.

One of the most memorable lines from any Adam Sandler movie that I can remember was in "The Water Boy" and came from a character named Townie. I heard this statement throughout the entire movie and it constantly brought a smile to my lips. The line was simply this:

"You can do it!"

I want you to understand that this quote is true for you today in your life. "You can do it!" I don't care where you've been or what you have been through—you can dig out. You can begin to live a life of purpose and watch your personal life improve and the lives of so many more in this world become improved because of the seed that has been planted inside of you. But you have to begin to believe it about yourself.

You are not insignificant. In fact, you are a person of great significance. Sometimes we begin to believe the lie that the world doesn't care about us anymore. We begin to believe that if we were no longer here that no one would even know the difference. There is no better movie that puts that into crystal clear perspective than the Christmas Classic, "It's a Wonderful Life".

In this movie there is a man who believes that his life is pointless and useless and of no value. Through a series of events he begins to realize that his life does have purpose and there was a reason for his existence. And in the midst of this realization, we hear these words spoken by the angel Clarence to the man questioning his purpose for life:

"Strange, isn't it? Each man's life touches so many other lives. When he isn't around he leaves an awful hole, doesn't he?" [3]

—**Clarence** *(Angel assigned to George Bailey)*

That quote was as true for the main character, George, as it is for you. Your existence means something and there is a great reason that you are here today. You are planted where you are for an express purpose. Maybe in this season there is something for you learn or people for you to meet. I don't care if you are sitting in a homeless shelter or in the Oval Office, you can learn something where you are. You can touch lives where you are. There is a great purpose for you exactly where you are right now. Embrace that purpose and begin to move forward.

Fulfilling the purposes of your life is no one else's responsibility except your own. Quit blaming your spouse or your boss. Quit blaming your past or those difficulties that you have faced in life. Quit blaming sickness or life situations. Quit blaming all together and say to yourself, "I am who I am because this is who I choose to be." For true change to happen, it has to happen with you wanting it. Embrace change and *become the change that you want to see in the world.*

3

The Sphincter: Getting the Crap out of Life

I still remember the early nineties and a duo that made their mark on American television in a skit show called "Saturday Night Live". There were two guys, a brunette and a blonde, who would sit on a couch and talk about music, life and girls—"Schwing!" These two guys were affectionately known as Wayne and Garth from "Wayne's World".

A movie was created in 1992 carrying the same name as this pseudo show from SNL and there was a conversation in it that I will never forget. It was between Wayne and a villain named Noah Vanderhoff. It went like this:

Wayne: A sphincter says what

Noah: What?

Wayne: A sphincter says what

Noah: What?

Wayne: Exactly!

It was the first time I ever heard of a sphincter, but for the next two years it was a staple in my vocabulary. It became a common jab amongst my friends and I would even play the 'sphincter says what' game with older people who had no idea about such great movie genius as "Wayne's World". The amusement behind the word was that many people had no idea what you were talking about. They were sphincter-ignorant.

Your body has many sphincters; in fact there are over 50 in the human body. The one which Wayne was referring to, however, sits at the threshold of the anus. In fact, there are two sphincters that sit by your anus which control the exit of feces from the body, an internal and an external. The former is involuntary while the latter is voluntary and they work together to keep you healthy.

Essentially, the sphincter is the doorway of crap. These are the muscles that push all of the crap out of your life… literally. Without these muscles, our bodies would be in grave danger. We would find all of the waste beginning to back up in our lives and, over time, a poison and toxicity would begin attacking our bodies from the piles of crap that were left behind.

Our personal lives are no different. We need to assure that there is a sphincter accessing the crap in our lives and causing it to exit our bodies and our minds. There has to be a doorway for the crap of our lives to exit out of. Because, if there isn't, than we will find an increased toxicity in our lives and damage that can eventually become irrevocable.

Just like the sphincters around the anus, there is an involuntary and voluntary response to the poisons that enter into our lives. There are certain things that our body automatically tells to get out and keep out and then there are other things that we have to take the lead on to assure that they depart from our lives. Our awareness and reactions to these poisons will allow us to live in a toxin free atmosphere.

INVOLUNTARY SPHINCTER REACTIONS

I will never forget my first hit of a cigarette in my early teens. It was a Virginia Slim Light 120, which is slightly emasculating to admit. Sneaking into my mom's pack, I had taken one of the thin, long tubes and a lighter. I was so excited to follow in her footsteps and can still remember how cool I thought she looked breathing smoke like a medieval dragon. I popped it in my mouth, set fire to one end and sucked through it like it was an extra thick milk shake. Spit and smoke flew from my mouth as I hacked and coughed and struggled for air. My body was violently rejecting the smoke that had entered into my lungs.

The next hit was disgusting, but not quite the same scene. I wasn't as ambitious with my inhalation and I took a smaller hit. I could feel a burn in my clean, pink lungs, but nothing like the first time. It was never again like the first time. My body had fought me in the beginning, but eventually bent to my will, allowing the smoke to come and make its home.

This same reaction happens with many foreign substances that make their way into our bodies. Sometimes it may be heroin and the sickness that is accompanied with it. The body will reach the point with heroin that the poison actually has a reverse affect and it rebels when the drug *isn't* there. The body is communicating that there is something foreign that is having an effect on it and that this effect is destructive. For others it is the consumption of too much alcohol and a worship session with a porcelain god. Their body is rebelling and getting rid of the excess alcohol before it has a lasting harmful effect on the body. There are many different examples of your body's involuntary sphincter reaction to negative influences on it.

The difficult thing about this is that our bodies will allow us to continue this behavior and correct us when things go too far… sometimes. Other times our bodies are unable to react in time and we find that our luck runs out and we end up having an overdose and dying because our bodies just couldn't take the abuse anymore. We end up taking a premature last breath because we didn't heed the warnings that our body was naturally giving us.

"To keep the body in good health is a duty… otherwise we shall not be able to keep our minds strong and clear."

—**Buddha** *(ancient spiritual teacher)*

All we have to do is think back to history in order to see lives and futures that have been stolen away by things such as drug and alcohol abuse, anorexia, cancer and many, many more. Many of us have personally been affected by people who have not heeded the warnings of their bodies… maybe even personally, by damage from not heeding the warnings of *our own* bodies. The great news is that it is not too late. The curtains have not closed on the performance of our lives… at least not yet.

Think about your life. What are some things that your body has rejected that you have continued to place in your body? Take a minute and write any things that come to mind here:

_____
_____
_____
_____
_____
_____
_____
_____
_____
_____
_____
_____
_____
_____

Now, at this point, you have decided that you are ready to do something about these toxins in your life. You recognize that nothing good is coming from these things. In fact, many times we have reached the point where we are no longer the ones in control of these toxins, but these toxins have now begun to control us. **The puppet is now pulling the strings of the puppet master and we are dancing to its music.** It is now time to break free from the control that these things are having on you.

1. Write down your intention and make it clear.

"I acknowledge that _____
(fill in the thing you want to be free from) has a control over me and I want to break that control. I will do whatever it takes to be free again."

2. Find specified support. For many of these things, there is a lot of control that has been taken over in our life and we are finding ourselves in a battle that we are unable to fight on our own. We need to find people who understand the struggle that we are in and want to stand with us and help us gain the victory. For many of us, we have been in this battle for years and it is going to take some time to dig out, but you need to find support so that you can break free. There are many different support organizations that deal with these different specific areas. Check out the website, **thebestmanifesto.com** for links to good organizations to partner up with.

3. Start today. The great lie that enters into the minds and lives of so many people who want to be free from negative holds in their life is simply, "I'll start tomorrow". Let me break it to you gently. . **tomorrow never comes!** Why? Because there is always another tomorrow and we find that this 'false hope' in some future remedy actually stops us from changing today and even has the potential to **keep us in** our toxic behavior.

4. Begin to learn. I want you to begin to learn everything that you can about the sticky web that you are finding yourself in. Read other people's stories about how they broke free. Read about the effects that your actions are having on your body and your mind. Watch documentaries that talk about the subject. Do everything that you can to become educated on where you are today and the potential damage that can happen tomorrow.

This knowledge will propel you to keep going when you feel like quitting. It will keep a fire in your bosom to change.

5. Talk about it. I need you talk about this with someone… anyone… everyone. The more people who can hear your story, the better off you are. By communicating your struggle to others, you will gain a greater perspective and understanding of yourself and where you are as an individual. Also, it will bring hope to others and take you out of the dark closet that many people find themselves in. When you commit to talk about your struggle, you are saying that you are not going to be held captive anymore. You are saying, 'I may not be where I want to be yet… but I sure as heck aren't where I was! And for that, I rejoice!"

VOLUNTARY SPHINCTER REACTIONS

There are other things in our lives that aren't necessarily as toxic, but we still need to address. There isn't an eminent death from their continuation in our lives, but they are still affecting us negatively. They may not be destroying us, but are propelling us towards a minimal existence and a less gratifying life.

These things make the difference between our achievement of the good, the better or the best in our lives. Many of us have good existences. Our bills are paid and we have a family and we think we know what we have in store for tomorrow. Others have taken their lives and made it better than it once was. Maybe these are individuals who had difficult childhoods or messy divorces or overcame trials along the way. Looking back they see that their lives are better than they once were. But, the purpose of this chapter isn't about simply getting you to a better life. It's about taking you to a new level altogether. It is about achieving THE BEST life that you possibly can.

"If you'll not settle for anything less than your best, you will be amazed at what you can accomplish in your lives."

—**Vince Lombardi** *(20th century football coach)*

I want to see you reach the point where you are living the best life that you ever had. I want to see you accomplishing things that you never thought were possible until now. I want your life to be an inspiration to millions. I want people who have no hope to find hope when they hear about your story. I want you to achieve THE BEST for your life.

In order to move from the good to the better to the best, you are going to have to become involved in the details of your life. You are going to have to join the fight for your todays and your tomorrows. You are going to have to take an honest look at where you are and where you are going and be willing to make some tough decisions about your current position. But before you know where you are headed, you have to know where you are. **Before you locate the destination, you need to find yourself on the map of your life.**

A great first step in locating yourself on the map of your life is to take a fearlessly honest and thorough look at your life as it is right now. I don't want you to remember how it was, because this will skew your view to either think you are better or worse than you once were. I don't want you to think of your goals or aspirations or where you are headed, because this will give you a false idea of where you are today. I want you to begin looking specifically at where you are today and asking yourself some tough questions. I need you to answer honestly. This is just for you. If you can't even be honest with yourself than you will never be able to achieve THE BEST life ever. Take some time to answer these questions.

Am I really happy right now? Why or why not?

_____

Do I feel like I know where I'm going in my life? Why or why not?

_____

What unhealthy habits do I see in my life?

_____
_____
_____
_____
_____
_____
_____
_____

Who in my life is pulling me away from my future goals?

_____
_____
_____
_____
_____
_____
_____
_____
_____
_____

Am I happy with how I spend my hours and my days? Why or why not?

_____
_____
_____
_____

_____
_____
_____
_____
_____
_____
_____
_____

What is one action that I currently do that I know is wrong but I keep doing it? Why do I keep doing it?

_____
_____
_____
_____
_____
_____
_____
_____
_____
_____

Name 3 time wasters that I do on a regular basis.

_____
_____
_____
_____
_____

_____
_____
_____
_____
_____
_____
_____

Name 5 things that I would like to see change in my life.

_____
_____
_____
_____
_____
_____
_____
_____
_____

Hopefully these questions caused you to think about some things that you hadn't wrestled with for a while. There are things right now that are stopping you from living THE BEST life that you possibly could. There are people right now that are holding you back from living THE BEST life that you possibly could. There are habits that you are holding on to that are stopping you from living THE BEST life that you possibly could. It is now your responsibility to activate the voluntary sphincter of our lives and say that you no longer want this poison in your life. Not because it is killing you, but because it is killing your potential and your future and the life that you were destined to live. Allow yourself to closely examine the four main areas of your life:

1. Physical: This is your body. Your flesh and bone. Physically, how are you doing in your life? Do you feel like you are making the most of the body that you have been entrusted with? Do you feel like you are working hard to maintain your health and vitality?

Write down some thoughts about your current physical condition:

_____
_____
_____
_____
_____
_____
_____
_____
_____

2. Mental: This is your mind. How do you feel about your current mental development? Do you feel like you are working hard in order to ensure that your mind is sharp and operating at its peak potential?

Write down some thoughts about your current mental condition:

_____
_____
_____
_____

_____
_____
_____
_____

3. Emotional: This is your emotional side. Are you happy... sad... enthusiastic... satisfied? How are you doing emotionally? Are you stuffing life down and becoming emotionally numb? Do you really "feel" life?

Write down some thoughts about your current emotional condition:

_____
_____
_____
_____
_____
_____
_____
_____

4. Spiritual: This is your spirit. Do you feel connected with a power greater than yourself? Do you feel like you are spiritually alive? Do you feel like there is an overwhelming awareness that there is more to life than just the temporal stuff that surrounds you?

Write down some thoughts about your current spiritual condition:

_____
_____
_____
_____
_____
_____
_____
_____
_____

All of these areas are very important for your overall health as an individual and your achievement of THE BEST life. We need to become whole, or complete, in every area of our life. We will often find one or two life areas strong while the others may be very weak. Our goal should be the active addressing of weak areas while maintaining the strengths that we currently have. We do this by inspecting areas in our life that we want to see changed. This is the first step.

Understanding what things we would like to see changed in our lives is not enough. We need to have a clear understanding of the *why* behind the *what*. Why do we need to get rid of this habit or person? Why do we need to change this action in our lives? Why do we need to refocus our lives? We must strengthen the reasoning behind our decisions.

Right now, I want you to make five different goals that you want to achieve that you believe would greatly improve your life. In this moment you are activating that voluntary sphincter and taking a stand against those things that are stopping you from THE BEST life ever. You are unwilling to continue in this same behavior and want to make a lasting change. Write down five goals that you want to meet here:

1. _____
   _____

2. _____
   _____

3. _____
   _____

4. _____
   _____

5. _____
   _____

Whenever we begin to develop a plan for our life, we need to understand two key components of the things that we are looking to change. First, we need to understand *what* things that we are looking to change. Then, after we determine what we want to change, we need to know *why* it is important to see these things change in our lives. The *why* is equally important to the *what* when it comes to lasting personal change.

You now have the *what*, but we need the *why* for the fortitude to keep going when the going gets tough. For each of these five goals that you just set, I want you come up with a minimum of five reasons *why* you want to see this change happen in your life. Feel free to write more, but you need a minimum of five different reasons why. Go ahead and get writing.

Goal 1:

_____
_____

Five reasons *why* I want to accomplish this goal:

1. _____
   _____

2. _____
   _____

3. _____
   _____

4. _____
   _____

5. _____
   _____

"A goal without a plan is just a wish."

—**Larry Elder** *(20th century American radio speaker)*

Goal 2:

_____
_____

Five reasons *why* I want to accomplish this goal:

1. _____
   _____

2. _____

3. _____

4. _____

5. _____

Goal 3:

_____

Five reasons *why* I want to accomplish this goal:

1. _____

2. _____

3. _____

4. _____

5. _____

Goal 4:

_____
_____

Five reasons *why* I want to accomplish this goal:

1. _____
   _____

2. _____
   _____

3. _____
   _____

4. _____
   _____

5. _____
   _____

> "Set your goals high and
> don't stop until you get there."
>
> —**Bo Jackson** *(20th century American baseball player)*

Goal 5:

_____
_____

Five reasons *why* I want to accomplish this goal:

1. _____
   _____

2. _____
   _____

3. _____
   _____

4. _____
   _____

5. _____
   _____

Now that you've written down the *why*s, I want you to make three simple action steps for each of these five things. They can be simple steps that you are going to take in order to assure that these changes take place. It could be as simple as "throw out those things that are making me have negative thoughts" or "tell her that I don't think it's healthy to see each other anymore" or "change where I hang out on Saturday nights". The simpler the better. Sometimes it is those simple actions that allow us to gain the momentum to have a true lasting change in our lives.

Goal 1:

_____
_____

1. _____
   _____

2. _____
   _____

3. _____
   _____

Goal 2:

_____
_____

1. _____
   _____

2. _____
   _____

3. _____
   _____

Goal 3:

_____
_____

1. _____
   _____

2. _____
   _____

3. _____
   _____

Goal 4:

_____
_____

1. _____
2. _____
3. _____

Goal 5:

_____
_____

1. _____
2. _____
3. _____

Excellent! Now make sure that you keep these goals close by so that you can look at your life every, day, week, month and year to assure that you are still stretching for your goals and directing your life in such a way that your personal sphincters are pushing all of that crap out of your life.

LIFE ENEMAS

This chapter is difficult for many because I am asking you to take an honest look at your life. Many times we just try to keep busy or maintain the volume of life so loud that we don't have to *deal* with those things that are truly holding us back. If you are reading this, then you didn't give up and you had the courage to face a lot of those dark areas of your life and I applaud you. You are well on the way to shaping your life into what you want it to be and moving toward achieving THE BEST life ever. And in order to keep this best life, it is important that you are continually keeping your finger on the pulse of your life.

As time goes on from this day forward, you are going to *experience* many different things. Life is going to come at you fast and there will be many mountain top experiences and there will also be many valleys that you will have to pass through. There will be highs and lows and seasons where you may feel like you've lost your way. You may even find different things that you have addressed in this book creeping back into your life. It is very common for old habits to try to reconnect to our lives even long after we have dealt with them. This is why I recommend a regular life enema every three to six months.

Allow this chapter to be your life enema. Whenever you are struggling or finding yourself being pulled from the best life to a good life, revisit this chapter. When you sense the struggle and feel tugged in different directions, come back to these pages to re-center. Or, when things are going great and you want to reiterate these goals into your mind, read over this chapter again and answer all the questions truthfully. You will find some areas disappearing altogether and other, new areas coming to the forefront of your life to be addressed. You will find a continual cleansing taking place as you come back to these pages.

The goal of an enema is to clean out the crap and to optimize your body's health. It is the same way with this chapter. You will find every area of your life—physically, mentally, emotionally and spiritually—being strengthened when you choose to examine, address and clean out the crap of your life. So, as they say in the doctor's office… "Let it flow!"

4

The Hands: "Stuff" of Life

There are five fingers surrounding the base of our hands and they prove to be the tools to touch, grab, feel and work. At the ends of our lives we will all look down at our hands. What will we see? Perfectly manicured texture, soft to the touch and free from scars or will we find hands that are cracked and used, filled with the stories of life manifesting themselves on flesh and bone? I want to choose the latter. I want hands that tell a story and share a legacy. I want flesh that has felt and that has been impacted by a life of purpose. I want the cracks of a fulfilled existence.

All of us have a decision to make when it comes to the 'stuff' of life and the activities that we do. Do we want to go for it and live a life of adventure or would we simply prefer to play it safe and make sure that we never put ourselves in harm's way? Are we willing to risk a crack or a scar in order to have the stories behind them?

Take an honest look at your life right now. Where are you? Are you just living the 'safe life'? Are you going through the monotony of day after day hoping that you can simply make your way through it without anyone noticing you? Do you find that you are being challenged and fulfilled? Do you find that you are excited to tackle each day? If not, maybe it is time to realign your life. What are the things that you are busy about? What are you doing with your time?

There was an Italian economist by the name of Vilfredo Pareto who helped us understand the correlation between time and accomplishment. His discovery came from land and peas. First, he discovered that in Italy, 20% of the people owned 80% of the land. Then, while studying a field of peas, he discovered that 20% of the peas produced 80% of the crop. These ideas flourished as he began to study the economic structure of other countries. His ideas eventually caught international popularity and became known as "the 80/20 principle". Simply, it means that 20% of our work produces 80% of our return on investment or 20% of your time is producing 80% of your value. Then, if you look at it the other way, 80% of your activity is producing only 20% of your results. Our goal for efficiency is to discover what activities are producing the greatest results and increase those activities while decreasing the useless ones.

According to this theory, our lives are filled with things that carry a minimal importance in getting us where we really want to be. Think about your average day and the things that fill your time. How important is filtering through that spam email or reading those Facebook status updates? How important is that lawn in comparison to those kids—how much one on one time is spent with each? How important is that car in comparison to that spouse? Why do you spend more time detailing it than you do talking about your spouse's day? What are the things that are taking up your time?

Can you identify five **TIME WASTERS** in your life? Write them down here:

1. _____
   _____

2. _____
   _____

3. _____
   _____

4. _____
   _____

5. _____
   _____

> "If time be of all things the most precious, wasting time must be the greatest prodigality."
>
> —**Benjamin Franklin** *(18th century statesman)*

Now, I want you to think of some things that you would like to see your time spent doing. Maybe it has to do with family or personal development. Quite possibly it could be doing that one thing that you've always wanted to do but never made the time for. Maybe it is reading or school or a hobby or sport. Write down five things that you would like to do in your life.

1. _____
   _____

2. _____
   _____

3. _____
   _____

4. _____
   _____

5. _____
   _____

I read a seemingly unassuming, small paperback book by Alan Lakein that radically changed my life when it came to my life productivity. The book is called "How to Get Control of Your Time and Your Life". Lakein is well known for his consultations about time management and the principles in his book are so profound that it is a must read for anyone truly trying to make the most of their life.

The simplified idea of the book stems from an individual allowing themselves to dream outside of the box about what they would truly like to do with their lives. But it is not solely examining life through a 'business' perspective, but really digs down to the core of what people really want with every area of their lives. Lakein encourages his readers to ask themselves three questions [1]. Let's work through these three questions together. Grab a notebook and keep it close in case you run out of space. Take your time and answer each question below:

1. What are your lifetime goals?

Take five minutes and write down as many lifetime goals that you can come up with. Dream big! Don't let your current life limitations stop you from really stretching and trying to imagine what you really want out of life. Think about your finances and family and education and health and relationships. Don't stop writing for five minutes. No answer is a bad answer. Ready… Set… Go:

THE BEST: A Life Manifesto

2. How would you *like* to spend the next three years?

Where do you see yourself in three years? Take another five minutes and apply the same advice that I gave you for the previous exercise. Don't stop till the time is up, and *no* idea is a bad one. Ready... Set... Go:

GP Hintz

3. If you knew now that you would be struck by lightning six months from today, how would you live until that moment?

You get the hint. Go ahead and let the ideas fly. You only have six months and life is going to end—so make sure that you make them really, really good! Ready... Set... Go:

_____
_____
_____
_____
_____
_____
_____
_____
_____
_____
_____
_____
_____
_____
_____
_____
_____
_____
_____
_____
_____
_____
_____
_____

I hope that you enjoyed this exercise and allowed it to bring the true goals of your heart to the forefront of your mind. When you start seeing a common theme or idea transcend from a lifetime to a three year to a six month goal, then you know that this is something that you are really passionate about.

Now, let's look at each of these three lists individually and rate your number one goal "A-1". This is the goal that gets you the most excited and the one that you want to see accomplished in your life more than any others. Next, you want to label an "A-2" (the second goal) and then "A-3" (the third goal). Now, do the same thing for your three year and your six month sheet and you will end up with nine goals that reflect your true heart and passion and what you really want out of life. From this point, Lakein helps you set up a plan for accomplishing these goals in your life.

You begin to:

1. List possible lifetime goals

2. Set priorities for your new A-goals.

3. List the activities for your new A-goals

4. Set priorities and identify A-activities

5. Schedule the A-activities

6. Do them as scheduled

For working this exercise further, I would truly recommend purchasing Lakein's book at **thebestmanifesto.com** and working through it. But, you have a great start. You have now discovered nine things to aim for and a direction to begin moving. Now let's take those nine things that we have and begin to develop them a little further.

For each of the nine things that you have chosen, let's write down five steps to achieve them. Some items may take less than five steps, but most will take five or more. Let's look at two practical examples:

Goal: Get a tattoo

Step 1: Decide where you want the tattoo to go

Step 2: Decide what the purpose behind the actual tattoo is (sentimental, funny, personal, etc.)

Step 3: Begin looking through tattoos that carry that theme

Step 4: Begin researching tattoo artists and find one that you appreciate their work

Step 5: Set up a meeting with the tattoo artist

Notice that we didn't reach the step of actually getting the tattoo yet. That is just fine. You will find that by simply taking the first five steps, the next five steps will be easier to plan and you will have some momentum that will take you in that direction. The hardest steps to take are the first ones. After you start moving in a certain direction, you will find yourself taking the steps easier each day. Let's look at another popular and not so clear cut goal:

Goal: Make a million dollars

Step 1: Clearly define *why* you want to make a million dollars (Purpose propels you. You can stay motivated easier if you have a clear cut purpose. Your motivation is going to be a lot different if you want a million to fill your mattress so you can sleep surrounded by the smell of money versus a desire to build five hundred wells for thirsty African children. Why do you want the money?)

Step 2: Clearly define *where* you are right now. What is your current financial situation? Write it down and firmly understand it.

Step 3: Understand your financial strengths and write them down. What do you know? Do you understand stocks and bonds or rental units or nothing at all? 'Know thyself'.

Step 4: Eliminate high interest debt. You are going to be treading the waters of life if all of your money is going out to satisfy high interest debt. Make a plan to eliminate this debt and attack it.

Step 5: Clearly define how much you would need to make in order to reach a million dollars in your allotted time frame and begin examining things that you can do to reach that million dollar mark.

I know that we aren't there yet with our plan, but if you have honestly worked through these five steps, you are well on the way to making your first million. The majority of people don't even go through the steps that you just did. Everybody wants to be rich, but no one wants to put in the work. The difference between you and them is that you just put in some work. And, as you worked through these five steps, I bet you were attaining wisdom and ideas about what your personal next step should be. You are thinking of different ways that you could earn money and discovering strengths that you have and how to use them to make money. Don't forget about the journey... it begins with a single step.

And in order to do any of these things we have to have a firm control over the time of our lives. Who is controlling your time? Is it a friend? a spouse? a job? an addiction? ...or you? It needs to be *you!* You need to be the one controlling the time of your life. We've taken a great first step in this time control by defining what we would like to see our life being filled with and the direction that we would like to be moving. But now we need to discover how to take back the control of our time.

We are the only ones who are responsible for how our time is spent... this ultimate commodity and great equalizer of life. We have the potential to invest the time of our lives and make great returns or squander the very minutes and hours that we are entrusted with each day. We have to know how this great commodity is being spent, invested or wasted in our lives. We need to know where we currently are.

Grab a pen and paper or your laptop because we are going to do some time investigation about our lives. I want you to take this paper or make a spreadsheet in one hour increments for a twenty-four hour period. Go from midnight at the top through 11pm at the bottom. Every hour I want you to have a few lines that are prepared to be filled in by you. (You can download a free spreadsheet at **thebestmanifesto.com**.)

Now, for a week I want you to record the 'highlights' of your life. How are you spending your time? How many hours are you sleeping, reading, watching TV, spending time with the kids or working on the car? Write down about how much time you spent on each thing. For example, if you watched a 30 minute episode and then played with the baby from 4p-5p on

Monday, then in parentheses put (30 minutes) next to each item. At the end of the week, I want you to calculate up the hours and put the total hours in some greater categories.

I recommend that you use the following categories, but you could add some of your own if you have specific areas that you are examining:

- Goal Pursuit
  (How much time was spent on pursuing any part of your nine goals highlighted earlier in this chapter?)
- Sleep
- Personal Care
  (showering, getting dressed, haircuts, etc.)
- Work
  (includes commuting, working and time spent preparing for your job)
- Faith
  (includes prayer time, religious activities and/or trips to religious facilities)
- TV time
  (This is a category of its own. I want you to know how much time you spend in front of the TV.)
- Personal Recreation
  (What are you doing to have fun and enjoy life?)
- Intellectual Pursuit
  (What are you doing to increase your intelligence and knowledge? Includes studying, school, conferences, etc.)
- Hobbies
  (Include time spent on specific hobbies that you enjoy.)
- _____
  (Make some categories that are specific to your life that you would like to keep track of.)

Now that you have a good specific picture of a week in the life of ME, ask yourself some tough questions.

Am I satisfied with how I am living out the hours of my life? Why or why not?

_____
_____
_____
_____
_____

Do my activities reflect my priorities and those things that I think are important? Why or why not?

_____
_____
_____
_____
_____

Is there a certain area that I am embarrassed by and what am I going to do to fix it?

_____
_____
_____
_____
_____

If I continue the way I'm living now, what may I be disappointed about?

_____
_____

_____
_____
_____

"Open up your eyes. Look within. Are you satisfied with the life you're living."

—**Bob Marley** (20th century reggae musician)

What are three things that I can change today about my schedule that will help me live out my goals and dreams?

1. _____
   _____

2. _____
   _____

3. _____
   _____

Our lives are our responsibility. We need to take ownership of where we are and where we are going. But what are we supposed to do when we find ourselves being pulled off track by the actions of another? What do we do when other people are controlling our time and dragging us down? Well, for these situations, we need to examine and implement some healthy boundaries in our life.

The concept of boundaries has become a popular one in our current culture. I like this definition that I stumbled across online:

"Boundaries are the emotional and physical space that we place between ourselves and others. Setting proper

> **boundaries is important to our mental health. When appropriate boundaries are not set, we run the risk of becoming either too detached from or too dependent upon others."** (2)

So, when we begin to examine how we are spending our time, boundaries will assure that there is a proper space between us and others. This space can move in both directions. Sometimes, we need to allow people to be closer than they are because we have pushed them too far away. But other times, we need to allow for a greater space so that others are not allowed to control our lives or dictate how we spend our time. We need to be the ones who are in control of our lives.

I can think of no greater work that covers this subject than the book written by Dr. Henry Cloud and John Townsend called *Boundaries: When to Say Yes, How to Say No to Take Control of Your Life*. (3) I would highly recommend the reading of this book if you find that your time is being controlled by others or if you would like to learn more about this captivating subject of 'boundaries'. For the sake of this work, I want to give you some quick steps to establish healthy boundaries in your life.

LET'S LOOK AT FIVE STEPS TO HEALTHY BOUNDARIES:

1. Know thyself: You are finding this to be a reoccurring slogan in this book and I think that it is one of the most important things that we can do in our lives. We need to know and understand our strengths and also our weaknesses. We need to have a firm understanding of whom we are and what we are struggling with. I need you to begin to understand yourself and why you are doing the things that you are doing.

2. Know thy enemy: The enemies in your life are those things and/or people who are stealing away your time. I need you to identify who or what is stealing away your time. They may not even know that they are doing it, but we need to become aware of these situations that are dragging us further away from the life goals that we have set.

3. Reinvent your vocabulary: There are certain words that I imagine you have a hard time saying. For example, "no" or "Sorry, but I can't" or "Absolutely not". Your lack of fortitude is causing you to get sucked into a lot of things that you don't want to be involved in and spending the days of your lives on projects or with people that you could care less about. I need you to begin to practice saying this one word: "**No**". Stand in front of a mirror and let the word roll off your tongue. Let it echo through the rooms of your house. Shout it from the rooftops and know that you are taking back control every time you say it.

4. Post a Sign or Leave a Message: Begin to communicate to people that you are taking time for yourself. Close the door to your office. Put up a sign saying, "Do Not Disturb... Will be Available at 1p" or "Out of the Office till Wednesday". Or, leave a message on your cell phone saying, "I will be busy until Monday morning. Leave your message today, and I will return it by Tuesday afternoon." Knowing that you have purposely expressed yourself through a sign or a message, you will not have to have the awkward conversations where you tell people that you are too busy for them. Let something else like technology be the bad guy for you.

5. Superglue Your Lips Together: OK, maybe that's a little extreme, but you need to learn that you don't always have to volunteer and/or say something. I want you to shake your head up and down, keep eye contact, plaster a big smile on your face, and don't say a word. You can listen and nonverbally support what someone is saying without becoming the person that has to take the project on their shoulders. Many times people are unwilling to pull the trigger and specifically ask you to do something. They are so used to you just taking it upon yourself, they never have to ask. So smile, listen and when the conversation ends, turn and walk away. You *don't* have to do everything that enters your eardrums.

Finally, I want to encourage you to not give up. You have a passion in your life. There is something that you are fired up for and this is the reason for your existence. It is the passion that gets you energized and excited about getting out of bed each day... this passion that rose to the top in the exercises in this chapter... this passion that we've been looking at... this is worth fighting for. *You* are worth fighting for!

Your tomorrows rest securely in your todays. That thing that you are doing today will dictate how your tomorrow will be. Do you want your tomorrow to be exciting and fulfilling? Do you want to be satisfied and happy with where you are and what you are doing? Or, do you want to simply be doing that same old thing day in and day out?

This chapter has been about examining and realigning our lives: What is really important to you and how you can assure that you are able to accomplish all that you want in your life. How can we make sure that the days of our lives aren't simply slipping by and leaving us with the regrets of a wasted life? I think the main way that we can ensure this is to make sure the areas of our life are in proper order. This comes back to our understanding of our lives and what is truly important and how we are going to spend our time.

I was at a conference once with a speaker who helped me understand this simple concept. He had two large jars on a table in front of him and he began talking about how busy every person in the crowd was and told us that the jars reflected our lives. He started talking about taking the kids to soccer games and emails to read and phone calls to return and all the house work that needed to be completed. He filled the first jar with small pebbles and sand which reflected all these things. He then talked about those real important things in our lives. He talked about the dreams that we had and the things that we longed to fulfill with our lives. He talked about passion and purpose and the BIG things in our hearts. He brought out three large stones and set them next to the jar and asked us a simple question, "How are we going to get the big things back into our lives?"

He tried to fit them into the jar with the sand and the pebbles in it, but there was no way that he could make them fit. He couldn't even get one to fit, let alone all three. So he turned his focus to the other jar... the empty jar.

"The only way that we can accomplish all that we need to in life, is by keeping our lives in the proper perspective" he said. "We need to take those things that are most important and add them into our lives first." He then took the three large rocks and placed them into the empty jar. "If we will put those BIG things into our lives *first*, then we will have plenty of room for all of the other stuff that we need to do." He then took the first jar filled with sand and pebbles and poured it into the second jar. All of the contents poured out over the stones and filled the jar up to the brim, but didn't overflow.

Sometimes we think that we need to focus on the endless pebbles and grains of sand in our lives first. This is all the busy work of life... but this is a grave mistake. If we instead turn our focus onto those BIG goals of our lives, we will find ourselves accomplishing all of those other things too; allowing both the stones and the pebbles to fit nicely into the jar of our life. So many of us are trying to cram our boulders into a jar full of sand when we need to be emptying out our jars of sand, placing our boulders in and then allowing the sand to fill in the cracks and crevices of those boulders.

Today, begin refilling the jar of your life. Take action and you will *never* be the same again. Get busy doing the most important things of life!

5

The Lungs: Breath of Life

The sun clipped through the window and bounced off the picture on the wall. It was bright and got stuck in my pupils as the photo slowly came into focus. I had heard the words before, but this time they sank deeply into my soul. I read: **"Life is not about the amounts of breath you take, but about the moments that take your breath away."** I smiled.

Those words had come into a greater perspective to me in the previous years. I had begun to live like this and truly desired to make my life count. I wanted to experience life and capture the essence of creation. I wanted memories to stack on top of memories and fill the volumes of my life. I wanted life to be interesting enough to write about, to talk about, to inspire.

I love the toast in the movie "Hitch". The question is raised, "What should we toast to?" and then you hear the main character, Hitch, say these memorable words:

"Never lie, steal, cheat, or drink. But if you must lie, lie in the arms of the one you love. If you must steal, steal away from bad company. If you must cheat, cheat death. And if you must drink, drink in the moments that take your breath away."

Ahhh! Yes. I understand. I want to jump on the table and shout at the top of my lungs, "Oh Captain My Captain!" as Robin Williams expounds on the importance of 'Carpe Diem' or 'seizing the day'. I still hear his words as he talks to his students about the great poets who made their lives count in the movie "The Dead Poets Society":

"They're not that different from you, are they? Same haircuts. Full of hormones, just like you. Invincible, just like you feel. The world is their oyster. They believe they're destined for great things, just like many of you, their eyes are full of hope, just like you. Did they wait until it was too late to make from their lives even one iota of what they were capable? Because, you see gentlemen, these boys are now fertilizing daffodils. But if you listen real close, you can hear them whisper their legacy to you. Go on, lean in. Listen, you hear it?—Carpe—hear it?—Carpe, carpe diem, seize the day boys, make your lives extraordinary."

These two words, "Carpe" and "Diem", still echo loudly in our hearts today. We first find their appearance in a Latin poem by Horace where he says, **"Carpe diem, quam minimum credula poster"** or **"Seize the Day, putting as little trust as possible in the future."** We find the poet giving us a command or a challenge to make the most of the day that is lying before us. He is giving us control to conquer and seize our days and to use them for our will. He is calling us to be proactive about our todays and live as if there was no promise of a tomorrow.

When we talk about the lungs and this breath of life, we are looking at how to take control and make our lives extraordinary. We are looking at how we can make our lives truly count and enjoy the life that we are living. We want to reach that place where we are excited about getting out of bed in the morning because we have a new day to conquer. We want to reach that place where we stay up late because we don't want the day to end. There is an overwhelming passion to be achieved in our life.

This passion and excitement can be found in the concept of spirit. Each of us is a person of spirit. Yes, we are flesh and bone and we have a mind, will and emotions. But the spirit is so much more. Spirit takes Man to another level and enables Him to sense and experience a greater level of life. We really find the spirit of an individual becoming the essence of who someone truly is—**this is the choicest or most essential or most vital part of an individual.** Our spirit is that place.

"Where the spirit does not work with the hand there is no art."

—Leonardo Da Vinci *(15th–16th century Italian artist)*

I have heard some say that "spirit" is "the breath of life". It is that thing which is bringing life and health and hope to each of us individually. I have met many individuals who seem to have everything going well in their life; they are strong and healthy and have money and loved ones around them, but are asphyxiated from their neglect of the spirit. Our lives must cultivate spirit and employ awareness to the health of our spirits.

For all of us, we have had moments that have taken our breath away. There have been times that we always go back to as "amazing" or "life changing"… in a good way. Some of us have to go all the way back to childhood or our teen years to find that memory. Begin to think about your life. Begin to go back to that good place.

Can you remember a time as a child where you were in the **"perfect place"** and you were filled with so much love and grace that you didn't want to be anywhere else? Do you remember a moment that a camera could have never captured what you were feeling in your heart? Can you remember taking a deep breath and saying, "God you can take me now"?

Right now, I want you to think back through your life and tell me a moment that took your breath away. It doesn't have to be extravagant, but it does have to mean something to you. It does have to stir up your spirit and your excitement for life. It does have to move you. Take some time and describe this moment to the best of your recollection. Talk about your feelings and what you were experiencing in that moment. Go ahead… take your time and write. Keep a notebook close in case you run out of space and need to keep writing:

_____
_____
_____
_____
_____
_____
_____
_____
_____
_____
_____

"Great men are they who see that spiritual is stronger than material force, that thoughts rule the world."

—**Ralph Waldo Emerson** *(19th century American poet)*

_____
_____
_____
_____
_____
_____
_____
_____
_____
_____
_____
_____
_____
_____
_____
_____
_____
_____
_____
_____
_____
_____
_____
_____
_____
_____
_____
_____

Hopefully that exercise allowed you to tap into some emotions that you may have not felt for some time. If your breathless moment just happened yesterday, then you are well on the way to living a fulfilled life. For many, however, it has been quite some time since you have felt that feeling. Now, we are going to truly imagine what it means to plan for some breathless moments.

In order to do this, I need you to completely step out of any limiting beliefs that you have. I need you to erase the word "impossible" from your internal vocabulary. I need you to be willing to dream like you've never dreamed and reach for things that you only thought could happen to "someone else" and never to yourself. I need you to develop some BHAGs for your life.

The idea of a BHAG made its debut in a 1996 article [1] written by James Collins and Jerry Porras called **"Building Your Company's Vision"**. BHAG was an acronym that encouraged people to think outside of the box. The acronym stood for a **"Big Hairy Audacious Goal"**. I have used this concept in both my personal and professional life; however for this sake of this book I think we need to revisit this acronym. I like the word BHAG, but let's change it up a little. I want you to come up with some

"BREATHLESS, HAIRY & AUDACIOUS GOALS"

I don't simply want you to make a goal that is *big;* I need you to set some goals that are going to take your breath away. I want you to develop some plans that have always sat deep down in your soul, but have been scared to make an appearance. A lot of times we are scared to visit these desires because we feel that if they don't come to pass… we are a failure. I propose that we fail if we don't bring them out to the forefront of our lives. They are there, planted inside of us to grow and blossom. We need to give them the sunlight and water that they need and desire.

I need you to dream. What is going to take your breath away? For some it might be swimming with the dolphins; for others it is swimming with sharks. For some it may be seeing

Michelangelo's Sistene Chapel; for others it may be painting homes for the impoverished in Mexico. For some it may be sailing around the world; for others it may be setting sail from your current dead end job to pursue starting a company that you've always dreamed of. The goals are as diverse as the people in the world. They reflect who you are and what you want to make of your life. I do want to give you some broad guidelines about these BHAGs however:

1. **They can't be attainable in your current situation.** If you can already achieve it... *just do it!* It's not a BHAG if you already have the capability to achieve it today. It only becomes a BHAG if you have to stretch and reach for it outside of your current situation.

2. **They all must require action.** For example, I don't want a goal like "I want to be famous". I want more detail. What do you want to be famous for? What is your idea of fame? What are you going to do with that fame?

3. **Details. Details. Details.** The more details you have the better. They will help you to move towards the goal. Don't confuse details with an action plan. I am not implying that you write down the steps you need to take to get there, but have lots of details about what the "there" looks like.

4. **Go Big or Go Home!** I want you to go for the gusto here. I want you to stretch those wings and reach for crazy stuff. I want you writing things that others would say were never going to be able to happen. This list isn't for them, this list is for you. You can do it if you simply try.

5. **Set failures and limitations aside.** I need you to set every failure that you have ever had aside. Forget about every one of them. Pretend that they never happened. Did you fail at a company start up? No! You just learned one way that

wouldn't work. Replace the word "failure" with the words "learning experience". Now, you are better prepared to take that next step and follow your passions toward some incredible BHAGs.

Alright, let's get started. I want you to list some Breathless, Hairy Audacious Goals that you want to accomplish in your life. I want you to write for a minimum of twenty minutes. Don't stop. Keep writing. Let one build off of another and no idea is too big. Allow your goals to increase in size as you begin to get the hang of it. Go ahead, set your timer, get that overflow notebook ready and get started:

_____
_____
_____
_____
_____
_____
_____
_____
_____
_____
_____
_____
_____
_____
_____
_____
_____
_____
_____
_____

THE BEST: A Life Manifesto

"Think little goals and expect little achievements. Think big goals and win big success."

—**David J. Schwartz** *(20th century motivational author)*

_____
_____
_____
_____
_____
_____
_____
_____

Ahhhh! How did that feel? Liberating? Empowering? Fulfilling? Many times people will gain a great sense of accomplishment and fulfillment simply from putting these goals down on paper. Even though not one has been accomplished yet, there is some great satisfaction simply from writing them down. And in all honesty, this is the single action that is preparing your goals for upcoming realization.

The closest idea of a BHAG list has recently become popular is the creation of a "Bucket List". Who can forget Jack Nicholson and Morgan Freeman sitting on the top of a pyramid in Egypt talking about the meaning of life in the movie "Bucket List"? Their goal was to experience life and all the breathless moments that they had always dreamed of. They end up coming to the realization that the greatest things in life aren't always those things that we experience, but who we experience those things with.

"Friendship is a single soul dwelling in two bodies."

—Aristotle *(4th century philosopher)*

We just took the time to make a list of experiences and things that we wanted to do. Oftentimes, however, these things take the place of cultivating the important relationships that lie all around us. How can we join these two things—people and experiences? How can we include others in those breathless moments of our lives? Write down the names of five people who deserve to be included in the breathless moments of your life.

1. _____
2. _____
3. _____
4. _____
5. _____

By simply writing down these goals and these people, you have set cosmic forces into motion. It is not my place to explain how all of this works, but to simply declare that the moment that we commit a goal or a dream to paper, something magical happens and these things begin to be drawn to us and, oftentimes, these things happen totally unbeknownst to us. We don't have to manipulate life or force these breathless moments to occur for them to happen.

I personally did this exercise many years ago and tucked my list away in some book. Years later I pulled out the book and the paper fell into my lap. I had forgotten about it until that point as I unfolded it and began to read. Much to my surprise, many of the things that I had written had come to pass in my life. There was one, however, that was so specific that I didn't even remember writing it until I read the words. They said: **"Plant a church from scratch."**

I looked back at the past three years of my life and I saw how my life had unfolded. I saw how the relationships that I had made and the difficult times at my job and the passions in my heart had all worked together, until the moment in 2010 when I planted a church from scratch that has grown and impacted people from all over the world. However, I forgot that I had ever written that goal. It is just the way that my life unfolded.

This is the same with you. Your life is unfolding before you every day. There are things that you have total control over and there are other things that you have absolutely no control over. But, you have to reach the point where you begin to believe that all things happen for a reason and that "all things can work together for your good." It doesn't matter if you know *how* certain doors became open or closed in your life. Your knowledge of *how* something happens doesn't negate the fact that it *did* happen and that it has the potential to be used for the power of good in your life.

THE DESTRUCTIVE POWER OF LIMITING BELIEFS

Sometimes the greatest enemy that we have in achieving these BHAGs sleeps in the same bed with us at night. No… I'm not talking about your spouse! I'm talking about you and the limiting beliefs that you have about yourself. The minute that you say, "I want to do this or that," your limiting beliefs will begin to try to tell you all the reasons that it can't be done. You will often hear things like:

"You're not smart enough to do that. Don't you remember the last time you tried?" *or:*

"It will cost too much money. You can barely pay your bills now." *or:*

"You really don't have the skills to make that happen." *or:*

"You're too old." *or:*

"You're too young." *or:*

"You're nothing but a dreamer who won't… (fill in the blank)"

No matter what your limiting beliefs are, you are the only one with the power to counteract the destructive force that they are having in your life. You need to become aggressive and active in moving your lives forward and regaining control over your thoughts, life, and the beliefs that you have.

I understand that many of your thoughts have been with you for a very long time and may be difficult to dismantle all at once. However, I do believe that the first step in counteracting the destructive force of limiting beliefs is to admit the possibility that they may not be true. Open yourself up to the rare chance that the limiting beliefs that you once held as true… aren't true at all.

THE BEST: A Life Manifesto

One incredible way to begin to change the thoughts that you have about yourself is to read the stories of people who have impacted the world in great ways. You begin to read about their "humanity" or "struggles" and discover that in spite of those difficulties, they were still able to do great things with their lives.

Michael Jordan didn't make his high school basketball team. This could have given him the limiting belief that he wasn't good enough to play the sport. How would basketball be different if there never was a number 23 leaping over defenders with the grace and ease of a gazelle?

Dr. Seuss was rejected by 23 different publishers before the 24th said, "Yes". I look back on the first book I ever read, *Green Eggs and Ham*, and think about how my life would be different if this limiting belief that "your writing isn't good enough" would have stopped him from moving forward.

Dr. Wayne Dyer spent his childhood in foster homes and orphanages, starting life from a place of rejection. How many people would have not been helped by this author, speaker and motivator if he would have embraced the limiting belief that this world didn't want him or care about what he had to say?

And the list goes on and on. Everyone who has ever accomplished anything great in their lives has had to go head to head with their own limiting beliefs. They have had to look deeply into the mirror and make a decision about what they were going to do with what they saw. Either they were going to see themselves through the eyes of limiting beliefs or they were going to see themselves through a state of possibility.

In your life, I want you to start to look at yourself through a state of possibility. As you read other people's stories and hear about the great obstacles that they had to overcome, begin to change the wording of those limiting beliefs in your life. For example:

Change **"I'm too old"** to…

"The famous artist Grandma Moses began painting in her seventies and didn't even become popular until she was in her eighties. She lived to be 101 and painted 25 different works of art in her final year of life. Her top selling painting sold for 1.2 million dollars. If Grandma Moses can do it… so can I. I am *not* too old… I am in the prime of my life and just getting started!"

Change **"I'm too young"** to…

"If Justin Timberlake could get his start at the early age of 12 and launch his career to the heights that it has gone to… I am definitely *not* too young to make something with my life. I will draw inspiration to work hard and believe in myself and watch something great happens in my life, too."

Change **(fill in a personal limiting belief that you have)** to…

(A real life story of someone who overcame that limiting belief. Now reword that limiting belief to its opposite and prepare a declaration that will completely change that limiting belief to a belief that empowers).

Go ahead and write one out for yourself:

_____
_____
_____
_____
_____
_____

COMBINING BHAGs AND AN EMPOWERED BELIEF TO FILL THE LUNGS OF LIFE

We now have everything that we need to begin our journey to a breathless life. We are well on our way to experiencing a life that we may have never imagined being possible. We are set up for success and have gained the ability to accomplish THE BEST and most satisfying things in our lives. Now we simply begin to walk it out.

As we take the next steps of life, it is important to leave the doors of life open to those BHAGs that you created in this chapter. Look for opportunities to see them fulfilled. When you sense the lies of limited belief whispering in your ear, make sure that you are gaining new stories of people who have overcome these specific limiting beliefs and apply their stories to your life. If they can do it... SO CAN YOU! There is absolutely no difference.

But sometimes life throws us a curveball. Sometimes things happen that seem to throw all of our plans or desires out the window. When these things happen, you need to trust that there is a greater plan and that every day of your life is leading you closer to your own personal destiny. Every moment is bringing you closer to your newly acquired BHAGs.

I experienced one of those curveballs when my mom passed away at the early age of 53 from a heart attack. I wasn't ready for her to go and, being an only child, I felt like a part of my world died that day she did. Luckily for me, she had taken the time to write in a journal that I had given her that asked her to answer different questions about her life, childhood and desires for the future. Once she passed away I started reading her words, penned in her hand and spoken from her heart. I came across a page that asked her about something that she always wanted to do and was never able to achieve. She wrote:

"I always wanted to visit the Eiffel Tower and go to the top of it. I never had the chance, but I wish I could have made it there."

Within two weeks, I had purchased my ticket to France, arranged to stay in a hostel and was on a plane to Paris. My life had been falling apart and I welcomed the opportunity to leave and be alone. I landed on French soil and made my way to the hostel. I found a room, slept and awoke the next day. I was heading to my sole purpose for the trip… I was going to the tower.

I saw it a few blocks away and moved faster toward its base. Reaching the bottom of this monstrous mass of metal, I bought a ticket to the top, entered into an antique pod and slowly started my ascent. Voices spoke around me, but my ears ignored their tones. I just sat and stared as Paris became smaller and I got closer to my destiny.

At the final stop, I took a step from the elevator and breathed in the cold air. I walked to the edge and viewing the beauty of Paris, I closed my eyes. This trip wasn't about it and it wasn't about me… it was about closure to a relationship that meant the world to me. It was about a vicarious realization of a goal not met. I wished that I had her ashes to dump out so that she could have realized her goal. I didn't. I only had myself and her memories.

Opening my eyes, I walked around the perimeter and made my way back to the pod and then back to the French soil below. I had now done my part.

I still remember the moment that I opened that book I mentioned earlier and my BHAGs fell on my lap. I had written them long before my mom's death and long before she had even penned the words in the journal that I had bought her. I hadn't ever discussed with her the goals that she never met or the regrets that she had from the past. But opening that paper, I'll never forget a goal that I had written on my BHAG list years prior:

"Go to Paris and see the Eiffel Tower"

I didn't go there with a BHAG in mind. I went there to mourn and to celebrate a beautiful life and a horrible tragedy. But there, in the midst of that beautiful tragedy, was a BHAG of mine coming to pass. Even in the midst of your sad and difficult times, the steps of your life can still be directing you towards life and hope and the realization of the deepest desires of your heart. In every moment of life, rejoice, for your lungs are still filled with the breaths of life that are longing to be taken away.

6

The Mouth: The Lingo of Life

Perched upon a hard wooden chair I sipped my latte and stared at the face across from me. We had worked together for some time, but things had quickly fallen apart. Now, our relationship—both professionally and personally—was coming to an end. I smiled with love and grace while reminding myself that I needed to control my tongue.

I had already communicated my thoughts on our professional relationship and clearly informed him of my feelings about our personal side too. Any more would have been hurtful and for the purpose of tearing down another to build myself up. There would have been no fruit toward healing or reconciliation… only the satisfaction of being right—which after a while becomes a lot less satisfying.

We parted in a good way and I can honestly say that it was the first time in my life that I had passed the tongue test. It was the first time that I had operated at a place where I was controlling my tongue and my tongue wasn't controlling me. I shook this man's hand, thanked him for the time that we had together, and walked away with my head held high. This is how we can leave confrontations and difficult situations if we know that we've controlled that tongue of ours.

There is a great saying that goes: **"The power of life or death lies in the tongue."** This muscle that lies touching teeth and gums has the power to build up or tear down... enhance or destroy. And even though it lies caged between molars and incisors, it sometimes will break free and has the power to completely destroy our lives.

"Many a man's tongue broke his nose."

—Seumas Macmanus
(20th century Irish poet and dramatist)

Our mouths can get us into trouble and the words we say have the power to destroy relationships forever. One hateful word has the power to obliterate a life-long friendship. A snide remark has the power to plant seeds of divorce in the heart of a spouse. A few juicy nuggets of gossip can get us fired from a great job. Our mouths can lead us through stormy waters or guide us into the rocks of destruction.

Like anything, the work of controlling our tongue will take a conscious effort and a lot of focus, but it is possible. Amy Grabiel of MIT's McGovern Institute has thoroughly researched the formation of habits in a person's life and has shown that the neurons in your brain actually change their firing patterns when habits are learned. Then, when a habit is "unlearned" (or changed), those neurons change again. What happens, however, when a person goes back to those "old habits"? Well, the neurons return to those old patterns and the habits return. [1]

This means that we have the power to actually alter how the neurons are firing in our brains by the actions that fill our day to day life. When it comes to our tongues, we have to begin to ask, **'What is coming out of my mouth?'**

Imagine if you were to carry a voice recorder with you all day that would start recording every time that it heard your voice. What would you hear? What message would the words out of your mouth send?

The words that are coming out of our mouths are conditioning us and are actually creating something. Are the words that we say leading us where we want to go or are they sending us in the wrong direction altogether? Are we getting conflicting messages from our brain and our mouth?

Do we hear ourselves saying things like:

"I don't know how to do that." *or:*

"I can't." *or:*

"I am just not qualified." *or:*

"She is a better candidate than me" *or:*

"I'm just lucky to have a job."

We could cover a million more and wouldn't even begin to scratch the surface. Each and every single day, people from all over the world are repeating a limiting **"I can't do it"** mantra that is hindering their abilities and their future prospects. It is like there is a CD playing in their heads each and every day filled with these limiting thoughts and beliefs of themselves. If we want to get control of our thoughts and lives, then we need to take that CD and use sandpaper to scratch and scratch and scratch its surface. It needs to be so scratched that it will *never* play the same again. We need to destroy those grooves so that we won't find ourselves going down that road believing those lies about ourselves anymore.

Then, when the old patterns have been destroyed, we are able to begin to rebuild the grooves of our lives. However, these grooves need to lead to new places and carry different messages than the ones before it did. And the way that we rebuild the grooves of life is to begin to believe a message that may even run contrary to what your mind has ever believed before. **We need to begin to address specific areas of 'weakness' in our thought patterns and begin to speak things *not* as they are (in our current minds) but as we want them to be (in our current lives).**

Historically, one way that has seen great success is the employment of "affirmations". An affirmation is simply the assertion that something is true. The trick is to find things that we want to be true in our lives that we may not thoroughly believe, but that we want to believe, and say them as if they are true.

A common mistake that I often see with people that use affirmations is that they are saying something that they already believe to be true in their lives and are simply agreeing with that belief that they already have. This is good… however for the purpose of reprogramming the patterns of our lives, we need to choose things that we don't believe to be true and begin to speak those things into existence. Let me give you some examples:

Current Thought: I don't think that I have the intelligence to go to college. I have always been told how dumb I was and that I'd end up just like my father working a dead end job.

Affirmation: I am smart. I can learn anything. With dedication, I can do anything I put my mind to. I can graduate college and the only one who has the power to stop this from happening is me.

Current Thought: I am ugly. No one would ever want to date me. I have so much baggage and everyone knows the things I've done. I'm just lucky to get whoever notices me.

Affirmation: I am beautiful. Grace rules my life. I have learned what I don't want from life and I know that I have great worth. I deserve the best. There is someone out there who will love me for me and is my perfect match. I refuse to settle for anything less than the best.

Current Thought: I am overweight and unhealthy and I'm going to end up just like everyone else in my family—dying of a heart attack before I'm 50. There's no use, it's written in my genetic code and this is simply my lot in life. I might as well just enjoy the delicacies of life while I'm still alive.

Affirmation: I only get one shot at this life and I'm going to make it great. No one will steal my life from me. I am not my father or my mother… I am myself and I will change the direction of my family forever. I will become a role model for my nieces, nephews and other family members and the physical "curse" over my family is going to end with me. Right now… today.

These are just a few examples of how to use affirmations to empower yourself and allow major changes to impact your life. Right now, I want you to choose three limiting beliefs that you have about yourself. What do you think you can't do? How do you see yourself? What have people told you that you'd never be able to do? I want you to write out your *current* thought about that situation and then come up with an affirmation specifically about that thought that you have.

Current Thought:

_____
_____
_____

Affirmation:

_____
_____
_____

> "Any idea, plan, or purpose may be placed in the mind through repetition of thought."
>
> —**Napoleon Hill** *(20th century American author)*

Current Thought:

_____
_____
_____

Affirmation:

_____
_____
_____

Current Thought:

_____
_____
_____

Affirmation:

_____
_____
_____

Now, I want you to take these affirmations and put them various places in your life. Some examples would be over the visor in your car, in your phone, on your computer as a screen saver, on a piece of paper in your pocket, written in lipstick on your mirror, tattooed on your forehead backwards so every time you brush your teeth, you can read it. OK. Maybe that last one is a little extreme. But, hopefully you are getting the idea. I want these things everywhere and within reach for easy access. You need to get your hands on these things and repeat them over and over and over again each and every day. And, you need to **say them** with your mouth **out loud**. Don't just read them in your mind, but let the words enter the atmosphere of your world. You will then be employing the muscles of your life and allowing yourself to **hear** as well as **say** them.

Then, when the affirmation becomes true in your mind and you believe the words that you are saying and would apply them directly to your life at that moment, file them in a notebook and make another one in the same way that you did the ones above. You will continue to build on these for the rest of your life, and you will witness amazing changes in your life.

THE RECORDER TEST

The next thing that I'd like to see you do is to invest in a pocket recorder. These can be bought for anywhere between $20–$100 dollars depending on the quality that you want and the budget that you have. There are more bells and whistles on the more expensive ones, but you need to start where you can start. Then, I want you to hit the little red button and record a day of your life.

When the day begins and you first hit that button, it is going to be really weird. You are going to feel like some super spy or something, but the only one that you are truly spying on is yourself. You are going to be very aware of everything that you are saying in the beginning, but as the day goes on, you will forget completely about the recorder in your pocket and you will begin just being yourself. This is what we are listening for. When your brain is on neutral, what is coming out of your mouth? What are you saying?

Later that night, when you get home, I want you to simply listen to your day. Fast forward through the hour long soliloquy of your boss or your non-talking bathroom breaks or your chomping away on an apple. But, I want you to listen very closely when you are talking to a coworker or a spouse on the phone or your kids. What is coming out of your mouth and how is it coming out of your mouth? What is your tone and what words are you using? If someone were talking to you in this manner, how would it make you feel? What would your thoughts be about this person?

This is going to be very hard for some of us. When we come face to face with the reality of our words, it can be very sad and even scary. Even though the words come out of our mouths each day, we often don't really hear them. This exercise will have you not only hearing them... but questioning them. Left with the unedited picture of your life, you will have to make some decisions for change. You have to begin to gain control over your tongue. Not only in relationship to yourself, but most definitely with others.

What words were you using with others? Are you choosing words and conversations that are building up or tearing down? Are you encouraging or discouraging? Are you pushing people towards a better life or are you pulling them away from one. What do your conversations with others sound like?

Sometimes we start to hear things like:

"Why would you even try something like that?" *or:*

"Don't you think you're a little too old for that?" *or:*

"Do you really think that even needs done?" *or:*

"Can't you think of something better?"

We find sometimes that we can become the wet blankets in the lives of others. We may find that we talk down to some people or become very condescending. We may find that we treat some people better than we do other people and we have to begin to ask ourselves why. The goal is to hear our voice, not through the ears of the one who is speaking, but through the ears of the one who is listening.

We want to make an effort to ensure that we are in the business of building up others instead of tearing them down. We need to become encouragers and not discouragers. The main way that we are going to do this is by controlling what comes out of our mouths.

Think back in your life about those people who have told you that you weren't ever going to amount to anything. Think about those people who said that you'd never make it. Think about those people who told you that you may as well quit trying because it's never going to happen. How do you feel as you think of them and their comments?

Now, remember those people that believed in you. Remember those people that complimented you and encouraged you to keep going and to reach for the next level of life. Remember those who told you to never quit and to believe in yourself. How do these thoughts make you feel?

All of these different situations bring emotions to your life. On one side, we become frustrated or sad or angry. On the other side we are grateful and excited and amped for life. We are where we are right now because of a lot of those voices that have come into our lives in the past. It is time to choose to become that voice in the lives of others. Which voice are you going to choose to be?

I believe that we truly want to be the encourager. We want to be the ones who are taking people to the next level. We want to be the fire in the bones of people to change the world in great ways. But, in order to be that person, we need to make sure that the way that we are communicating with people reflects that heart and desire. And in order to do that, we are going to go back to our recorder.

Now that you've addressed some of the areas of your daily communications, I want you to do another day with the recorder in your pocket. I want you to go about the same activities that you did the first time. For example, if the last time was a Saturday at home with the family, do that again; or if it was a Monday at the office, repeat this. But this time you are going to make a conscious effort to become the voice or encouragement and life.

SHUT UP AND SPEAK UP

The quickest way to become the voice of encouragement and life is to simply shut up or speak up. With the recorder in your pocket, I want you to go through your day and every time that you are in contact with another person, ask yourself—should I **shut up** or **speak up**?

> Some coworkers are trying to drag you into some office gossip about the boss and the new secretary… **Shut Up**
>
> Your wife made a dinner that is lacking taste and you know you could have done a million times better… **Shut Up**
>
> Your boss is thinking about taking up a hobby which you are very familiar with… **Speak Up**
>
> Your teen got a B in a very difficult government class and she brings you home the report card… **Speak Up**

And the situations will continue to unfold all around you. The simple question to ask yourself is**, "Should I shut up or speak up?"** If what you are about to say is going to lessen the value of the individual or situation, then simply shut up, walk away and get out of there. On the other hand, if you have the opportunity to improve someone's worth or belief in themselves or their job, simply speak up and bring value to them.

THE BEST: A Life Manifesto

I still remember a time in my life when someone chose to 'speak up' and it changed my life forever.

"I know you can do it." His voice exuded confidence and belief for a person that didn't even believe in their own abilities... and that person lacking confidence was me.

"Uh... I don't know... I've never—" He cut me off.

"It doesn't matter. You can do it. They will listen to you."

I was being asked to do something that I had never done before. I was being asked to speak in front of people... a large group of people. I had heard the old adage about public speaking where more people would want to be in the coffin than read the eulogy. I was feeling like the dead man ready to be buried. I wanted to run away and hide, but the belief in his eyes made me want to believe in myself.

"Do you really think I can do it?" I asked with my eyes pinned to the floor.

"Look at me." His eyes now shone bright like the glare off of Captain Picard's head. *"I think that you are going to do great and I think you have something that people need to hear. I believe whole-heartedly that you can do this or I wouldn't have even asked you."*

Dragging my pupils from the carpet I looked at him. "OK. I will do it."

Since that first time public speaking I have spoken in front of thousands of people from all over the world. But I know that I never would have done any of it if it wasn't for that one person who believed in me and used his mouth to encourage. For that, I am eternally grateful.

THE LINGO OF LIFE

To truly begin living this out in our life, we need to actively pursue the lingo of life and not death. We need to understand that we make a conscious choice every time we speak to bring life or death. We choose to encourage or discourage. We choose to resurrect or kill.

We bring life into people and situations in three specific ways:

1. Shut Up! There is no quicker way to bring death or destruction than to practice the ancient art of gossip. Gossip is a destroyer and ruins everything pure about relationships. It breeds distrust and malice and hate and envy. It tarnishes the most beautiful things and spreads like an Arizona wildfire.

"Who gossips with you will gossip of you."

—Irish Saying

In life, we reap what we sow. Call it karma or the Divine Law of Retribution. If you choose to tear others down, then you will be torn down by others. What we give comes back to us. We need to make every effort to build up and never tear down. If we find ourselves being pulled into the world of gossip, we need to turn and run. Nothing good will ever come from gossip.

2. Speak LIFE over people! This is something that Mama taught you many years ago—**"If you don't have something nice to say, then don't say anything at all."** This is the equivalent of life and death. Choose to encourage and uplift. Choose to speak good things over people. Even if they don't have many good qualities, search for something good to say. At the very least… try some of these:

"You have a nice smile." *or:*

"You sure have had a rough life, but you still keep fighting." *or:*

"A lot of people have given up on them, but I still think there's hope." *or:*

"I've met a lot of people, but there's something special about you."

When you are around them, be an encourager. Let them know that they can do it. Let them know that you see that they are trying. Speak truth over them… maybe not the way that they see it, but the way that you see it. Let them know that they will get there and that they can do it if they just keep trying. Think of your words as an electroshock that is bringing their soul back to life.

3. Speak *life* over yourself! This is probably the hardest things for some people to do. I have met so many people who look at me and say, **"I believe good things about other people, but I have nothing good to say about myself."** They have been torn down so much, whether externally or internally, that they see no hope in their lives and no worth at all in themselves. In all honesty, if we can't speak life over ourselves, we are going to have a very difficult time speaking life over anyone else.

"I don't like myself, I'm crazy about myself."

—**Mae West** *(20th century American actress)*

How do we get to the point where we are "crazy about ourselves"? The steps are very simple. You can begin to notice the things that you are good at and let yourself know that you have skills and gifts and talents. After that, begin to take those areas that you would like to see improved and employ the affirmation technique that we discussed earlier in this chapter. Finally, begin to carry yourself as a person of great worth. You are a person of great worth and you need to carry yourself that way. Employ some swagger and watch what happens to your confidence.

This process of dealing with our tongues is a life-long one. You will always be working in this area. The goal, however, is to start today. Every day you are going to be learning things about yourself and developing in this area, so you might as well start right now. Take the tools that have been given and begin to use them, think about them and teach them to others. You will find that as you do these things, your life will begin to dramatically improve in every area and you will begin to taste the very sweetness of life.

7

The Brain: Mental Development

I don't know what it was that attracted me to him over all the others, but every time I watched the movie I couldn't wait for his appearance on the big screen. Maybe it was the way that he fell off that pole, losing some of himself all over the ground. Or, quite possibly, it was the wonderful song that he sang, as he poured the desires of his heart out to a young girl and her pooch.

> "I would not be just a 'nuffin
> My head all full of stuffin'
> My heart all full of pain
> I would dance and be merry
> Life would be a ding a derry
> If I only had a brain"

Of course I am talking about the scarecrow from the 1939 classic *The Wizard of Oz*. I can think of no better example of how many people feel today. Here you have an individual who feels like he is never going to be smart and that he has to go see a certain person in order to attain a brain. What he finds out at the end, however, is that the one thing that he didn't think that he had, was with him the entire time. **(I hope I didn't ruin that suspenseful ending for you.)** It is the same way in our lives.

You may even be reading this book right now and feel the same way as the scarecrow. **"I'm dumb"** or **"I'm just an idiot"** or **"I'm not the sharpest crayon in the crayon box"**. You've been carrying these thoughts around in your life for years now and have come to simply accept them as truths. In your mind, since these thoughts have become truths, they have now become facts and paint the reality of your current existence—and have imprisoned you.

I am writing this chapter, however, to pull back the curtain on the wizard. I am penning these words in the hope that you will reach the point where you abandon this false idea—that you are lacking intelligence or the ability to exercise wisdom in your life. No matter where you are today, you have the ability to gain knowledge and make an incredible impact on this world. And this impact will often come into a greater clarity when we begin to gain a better understanding of our most undeveloped assets… **our brains**.

At its simplest level, the brain is the boss of the body. This "leadership role" covers many different areas from causing your lungs to take in breath to remembering the combination to your gym locker. It has the power to remember and forget and solve problems and bury problems and equate emotions like joy or sadness to people, places and things. It provides decision making skills and walks you through everything from whether to watch a movie or not to choosing your future spouse. The brain is active in every part of our lives.

At a strictly biological level, the brain is made up of four major divisions. *"For "headier" studies—pun definitely intended—the biological structure of the brain can be broken down a lot further. But for the sake of this chapter, I want you to have a brief overview, not a job as a*

THE BEST: A Life Manifesto

neurosurgeon." These four major parts have specific functions which translate into the life that we live each and every day. Let's look at an overview of these four divisions:

Cerebrum: The cerebrum makes up the greatest part of the actual brain and has control over the body's voluntary muscles. In fact, 80–85% of the brain is made of up of the left and right hemispheres of the cerebrum. This is the "thinking" part of your brain. **This is the part of the brain that causes you to become a master champion at your favorite video game and how you can remember all the parts to the dance from "Napoleon Dynamite".** You may have heard the "right brain" vs. "left brain" debate in your life. This is in reference to your cerebrum. There is an understanding that your cerebrum is made up of two halves and there are scientists who believe that the right half helps you think of abstract concepts and causes you to be gifted at music, art, colors, shapes, etc. while the left enables you to be better at analytical things like math, logic and speech. Either way, your cerebrum is the part of the brain that is responsible for all of these different areas.

Diencephalon: Now don't get intimidated by this word. Very simply, this is the part of the brain that is underneath the large cerebrum. Located in this division of the brain are the right and the left thalamus, the hypothalamus and the pituitary gland. The hypothalamus sits right at the center of all the action and is known as your body's inner thermometer. **The last time that you worked out or ate some spicy food, what happened? You probably started sweating and this was triggered by the hypothalamus which was cooling your body down through sweat.** The pituitary gland is tiny, like the size of a pea, but very important. Its job is to produce and release hormones to your body. Have you ever known a kid that outgrew three pairs of shoes in one year? This was because the pituitary gland was doing its job and those hormones were causing those feet to grow in size.

Cerebellum: This is not to be confused with the cerebrum, though it is similar. Like the cerebrum, the cerebellum is broken down into two hemispheres, the left and the right. This part of the brain deals with muscular movements, and helps to maintain proper posture, equilibrium and muscle tone. It is at the back of the brain and is about 1/8 the size of the cerebrum. In addition to controlling the muscular movements, the cerebellum is vitally important to your balance. **If you were to watch the X-games and observe the most amazing skateboard trick ever, you can assure yourself that the greatest asset to the trick was the cerebellum which enabled the skater to keep their balance and land that amazing feat.** The cerebellum keeps us upright and moving along from day to day.

Brainstem: This part of the brain is positioned beneath the cerebrum and in front of the cerebellum and connects the rest of the brain to the spinal cord. It is responsible for all of the functions that are necessary for your body to stay alive, from breathing air to digesting food to circulating blood. It is in charge of the involuntary muscles inside of your heart and stomach and is in constant communication with the rest of your body. **It is the part of the brain that tells your heart to pump more blood as you are biking up that really steep hill or to start digesting that jalapeno and goat cheese quesadilla that you just ate.** If that wasn't enough, the brainstem also works like the brain's secretary by sorting through the millions of messages that are coming into your brain and dispersing them accordingly. It helps to make sense of our lives and provide our brains with the order necessary to produce maximum efficiency.

"The human brain starts working the moment you are born and never stops until you stand up to speak in public."

—**George Jessel** *(20th century singer, actor, director)*

Now that we understand the grand scheme of how the brain works, what does that actually mean for your life? How can you take the life that you are currently living and increase the knowledge and brain efficiency to produce more in your life? The great news is that you have the power to actually increase your brain's efficiency and to become smarter. This, however, will take some work on your part and may actually cause you to change some of your actions, but this change will produce a greater intelligence and will be well worth any inconvenience.

If you are serious about creating a lasting change in your life, I need you to never forget one of my favorite quotes:

"If you do what you've always done, you'll get what you've always got."

—**Mark Twain** *(pen name of 19th century American author and humorist)*

If you continue in the same way that you are today, you will never be able to bring about a lasting change in your life. You will never be able to accomplish all that you want to in life if you are unwilling to try new things and to get rid of some old things that aren't helping you in your current situation.

Don't listen to the words of Homer Simpson who said, **"How is education supposed to make me feel smarter? Besides, every time I learn something new, it pushes some old stuff out of my brain. Remember when I took that home winemaking course, and I forgot how to drive?"** I promise you that new information will never push out old information. In fact, new information is necessary for us to even keep the knowledge that we currently have.

Some people may think, **"Well, I'm just fine where I am today. I'll just do nothing because I have all the knowledge that I'll ever need to live my life."** This, however, isn't true when it comes to your brain because it works like a car that is moving uphill. As long as you are pressing on the gas, you will be moving forward. You might not be moving that fast, but you will consistently be getting closer to the top. If you put that same car in neutral, your car will not be simply sitting in the same place. In fact, it will begin moving backward and the longer that it is allowed to move in that downward direction, the faster it will go. Your brain is the same way. If you choose to sit around and do nothing with your brain function, you will begin to forget all that you have ever learned and you will progressively grow dumber and dumber. This is because of our ability to create neurons.

"Stupid is as stupid does."

—**Forrest Gump** *(character played by Tom Hanks in the movie "Forrest Gump")*

Neurons are brain cells that communicate with each other. When you made your grand entrance to this world, you had over 100 billion neurons which were primed to make their impact on humanity. As life goes on, these neural networks reorganize and reinforce themselves in response to different stimuli that enters into their world. According to the Franklin Institute:

"A healthy, well functioning neuron can be directly linked to tens of thousands of other neurons, creating a totality of more than a hundred trillion connections—each capable of performing 200 calculations per second. This is the structural basis of your brain's memory capacity and thinking ability" [1].

Throughout your life, it is important to maintain the creation and the interconnectedness of these neurons to enable the greatest intellectual potential of your life. Increased mental activity will ensure the stimulation of the creation of new neurons in your life and also increase the interconnectedness of these existing neurons. Think about it, by exercising your mind you are creating a stronger mental web to capture and produce greater intellectual insight, thoughts and ideas. But, like any muscle, your brain needs to be exercised to grow in strength.

And it is often the simple things that we could do that will greatly improve our lives and our intelligence. I want you to start with simple things that are going to cost you a minimal amount of money and time which will give the greatest return in every area of your life. I want to present you with some ideas. This is clearly not an exhaustive list, but here are some ideas to spark that gray matter for some goals that you can set personally.

Learn something new. Pick a subject that you have always been interested in and commit to learn it. This could be anything from learning a foreign language to dog grooming. There are innumerable resources available for you to learn all that you can about a subject of interest. In the beginning, most of these resources are absolutely free. If you enjoy it, take your education to the next level and pay for classes or books that will take you further into your area of interest. But, for right now, just get your feet wet. Learn something new and watch that brain activity increase!

Memorize names. Set a goal of memorizing the names of people in your life. Maybe you are a teacher of a classroom of students… commit to memorize each of their names. Or, maybe it is the coworkers that you just see in the break room each day. Make a special point of asking them their names and then commit those names to memory. Use little hints to help you. For example, if you work with a George, Paula and Harry you could see them in your mind as "George of the Jungle" **("Watch out for that tree!")**, "Straight Up Paula" **(Paula Abdul's most famous song)** and "Hairy Harry" **(because of that obnoxious Hemingway-like beard of his).** You have to make it personal and something that you are going to remember. Try it out. You can even work personal jokes into your conversations where you look at Paula and say, "Straight Up Girl" every time she says something you agree with. Or… maybe not.

Sing to solve problems. This idea brings the "right brain/left brain" concept to the forefront again. You could have a problem that you have been thinking about and don't really know what to do to solve it, so you decide to sing about it—hoping to discover a solution. You could simply be driving around in your car and singing at the top of your lungs about the problem. Or, you could get a song that just had a track with no words and sing or rap about the solution. You could just let loose and see what happens.

Record stuff and listen to it. There could be major issues at your job and you are having meeting after meeting about them. These meetings will often blur into one another and you walk away with only the highlight reel in your head, and you overlook some great ideas and nuggets of truth that are nestled in the midst of the discussions. Buy a recorder and record the meetings. Then, on your commute to and from work, listen to these meetings over again with the purpose of gleaning a greater understanding of the problem and working closer to the solutions. Also, you will find that this will generate fresh ideas in your mind as you are listening to yourself from a third person perspective.

Record yourself talking about life. This takes our recorder and allows us to use it in an active role for thought creation and not simply as a passive observer. It will allow you to speak ideas aloud and capture them on your recorder. Each day, take a different subject of your life and tackle it. For example, you can start each day with a question like "How can I make more money this year?" or "How can I be a better mother?" or "Am I really happy with my life?" Then, just let yourself talk about this question. You will be amazed about some of the things that will come up and some of the great advice that you have to give yourself about these different areas. Begin to deliver advice to your most important client—yourself!

Read or listen to books. Increase the amount and variety of ideas that you have coming into your life. Read or listen to books. I am a strong proponent of both. I used to only read non fiction, but now I see the benefit of a healthy balance between the two, non fiction and fiction. I think that there is a great advantage in the consumption of fiction books; however I think that far too many people spend all of their time reading pulp fiction when they should be devoting some of their reading time to educating themselves. A great tool that has exponentially increased the amount of book reading that I do in my life is the use of audio books. I take advantage of them every time I'm in the car, going for a walk or simply trying to fall asleep by listening to audio books. I always look for books that are "unabridged" so that I know that I am getting the exact same content that I would if I were reading the book in its entirety. The best place that I have found to get my audio books is at **audible.com.** You can become a member and get a great discount and a regular influx of stimulating books to add to your collection.

Get some sleep. I cringe at putting this in this chapter at the thought that some would use this advice to sleep their life away or take a daily nap when they should be out there positively impacting this world; however, I can't escape the facts. A brain that is sleep deprived does not operate at the same level as a brain that has had a proper amount of sleep. A professor of neurology at the University of Minnesota Medical School by the name of Mark Mahowald warns that any amount of sleep deprivation will diminish mental performance. He says, **"One complete night of sleep deprivation is as impairing in stimulated driving tests as a legally intoxicating blood alcohol level".** [2] So, make sure you're getting a proper amount of sleep to be operating at a full mental capacity.

Eat right. There is a universal understanding that how we eat affects our bodies. If you eat nothing but double cheeseburgers three times a day, your body is going to be affected by that diet. But something else that we need to understand clearly is that our minds are also affected by the diet that we consume each and every day. In fact, a study at the Harvard Medical School proved this idea. A group of researchers examined the data from more than 13,000 Nurses' health study participants who were aged 70 and older and found that the women who ate the most vegetables, especially green leafy vegetables (like spinach and romaine lettuce) and cruciferous vegetables (like broccoli and cauliflower) experienced a slower rate of cognitive decline than did the women who ate less vegetables [3]. Scientifically, there is a direct correlation between what enters your mouth and what takes place between your ears. If you want to increase your brain function, choose the right things to eat.

These are just a few different ideas of some steps that you can take to increase your brain function. Now comes the moment when you look specifically at your personal life and ask some tough questions. I want you to grab your pen and honestly answer these questions:

Do I want to be smarter and operate at a greater intellectual level? _____

Why do I want this for my life?

_____
_____
_____
_____
_____
_____
_____
_____
_____
_____
_____
_____

Don't forget the common theme throughout this book. The **why** will always motivate the **what**. If you don't know **why** you want something, there is a very low chance that you will ever actually achieve that thing that you are after. So, revisit the why section again and make sure that you answered it thoroughly.

Now, let's enter into that head ours…

Name three things that you are going to start today that have the potential to dramatically increase your intellectual capacity. As you list each thing, I want you to write why you chose that thing specifically and how you are going to assure that this action will take place.

THE BEST: A Life Manifesto

1. _____
   _____
   _____
   _____
   _____
   _____
   _____

2. _____
   _____
   _____
   _____
   _____
   _____
   _____

3. _____
   _____
   _____
   _____

Now I want you to make a commitment to yourself. I want you to really think about this commitment and why it is important to you. Think about what the benefit will be to you, those who care about you, and ultimately the world. Read this next paragraph and if you are serious about bringing about a lasting change, I'd like you to sign this commitment. But, I only want you to sign it if you are serious.

I am committed to assuring that I am continually challenging my current level of thought, knowledge and understanding. I am committed to growing my brain and using that increased knowledge for the betterment of this world. I will never stop learning. I will never stop believing that I have the potential to do anything I put my mind to. And, finally, I will never give up on myself. My future is worth an investment in my today.

Signed: _____

I want to leave this chapter with a quote from my favorite bear… Winnie the Pooh. He said this:

> "If ever there is a tomorrow when we're not together… there is something you must always remember. You are braver than you believe, stronger than you seem, and smarter than you think."

—**Winnie the Pooh** *(Character created by author A.A. Milne)*

From my heart to yours… ditto!

8

The Eyes: A Window to the Soul

I still remember the year, 1995, and driving around in my Ford Tempo with the windows down and my new CD playing loudly through the speakers. I was singing the chorus at the top of my lungs as the wind cascaded over my freshly shaved head.

> "Eyes wide open, I can't see
> Eyes wide open, what you mean
> Eyes wide open, I can't seem to be
> My eyes wide open, I can't see
> Eyes wide open, what you mean
> Eyes wide open, I can't seem to be"

John Rzeznik, the lead singer from the Goo Goo Dolls, was singing the cry of my heart on the song "Eyes Wide Open". I totally understood this idea of thinking that my eyes were open but being unable to see or understand. I was lacking any sort of vision for my existence and was simply living day to day and waiting for the roof of my life to collapse.

I was only 18 at the time, so I guess that I was in the place of many young adults, smoking up the ambition of my life while dreaming of a pretty and posh future. Personally, I was coming off the heels of a rough few years and was absolutely drained physically and emotionally. I just wanted to blow off steam and forget about life, but there was still this desire to understand the direction of where I was going. There was still this desire to have my eyes wide open.

I believe that there are many people out there who are in this same precarious position. They feel like their eyes are wide open and they are unable to see. They want to know where they are going and for what reason they are headed there… but that knowledge seems to elude them, dipping behind the dark corners of life.

OUR EYES ARE SENDING A MESSAGE

Oftentimes, the very thing that we use to physically see, our eyes, can communicate to others a very strong message about who we are and what we want. For example, have you ever met someone who wouldn't look you directly in your eyes? What kind of message did you get from that person? Or, what about someone who was staring at you with their eyebrows furrowed and crow's feet etched accordingly? What did you begin to think about that person when you noticed them? Or, what about that woman who is flirting with you and calling you into her vicinity from the other side of the room? She is communicating solely with the two orbs placed in her sockets. She is wooing you with only her eyes.

The eyes have an incredible power over our lives and those doors that are opening and those that continue to slam in our face. Many of us may have lost opportunities because of the message that is coming off simply from our eyes. The interviewer may have loved what we had to say and our resume, but our eyes were communicating a message contrary to the pen marks on the paper. Or, first dates have transformed into last dates because of how we chose to communicate with our eyes.

The effect that our eyes have on our lives is not solely external either. In fact our eyes are communicating internal messages to us each and every day. There is a transformation that is taking place inside of us because of what is entering into our lives through our eyes. We have an incredible opportunity to transform what is taking place internally and externally in our lives simply by taking a greater control over our optics.

There is a great old adage which says, "The eyes are the window to the soul". This is the picture that eyes let us see and communicate to other people who we really are. Not the plastic façade that so many of us put up on a regular basis, but who we truly are as individuals. In some ways, the eyes are not only the frame for others to see who we really are, but the door to our personal development and formation.

OUR EYES ACT AS THE GATEKEEPERS

I like to think of our bodies as castles that we have created. They are a place of refuge for us and for others. They can be strong and a beacon of hope for all those around us. And, in the castle of our lives, we have a gigantic door that can be lowered whenever we want. This door is the entrance for all that we allow to come into the castle of our life. The doors of our lives, in many ways, are our eyes.

We make the decision of what is worthy of entering into the castle of our lives and what is not. We have total control of what is taking place. Unfortunately, many of us just leave the doors of our lives down all the time and we are finding that a lot of unsavory things are entering in and beginning to destroy our castles… and ultimately our lives.

Imagine a fortified castle where the door is just continually open. Unsavory individuals would come with ill motives and find nothing stopping them from entering in. They come to steal your things and wreak havoc on those who call your castle home. They come to rape and pillage and have **their** way in **your** castle. They cause uneasiness and fear and an overall unhappiness. You allowed these individuals in by not manning the door of the castle. You are responsible for the castle door and if you are not doing your job, the overall castle of your life will be destroyed.

Our eyes become those gigantic front doors of our lives. We are the ones that have control over whether these gates are being manned or left wide open. We have the authority to say what it entering into the castles of our lives. Far too often, we are just living our lives with these doors wide open, letting anything and everything into the castle of our mind and life. And these "unsavory" things that we are letting into our lives are beginning to destroy us.

> ## "Keep guard over your eyes and ears as the inlets of your heart..."
>
> —**Anne Bronte** *(19th century British novelist and poet)*

A great example of one way we leave the front doors of our castles wide open is by setting absolutely no standards or stipulations on the things that we allow into our lives through the media. We will just allow any new blockbuster or television series to be consumed without setting any guidelines as to what our personal standards may be or to what we are allowing into our lives.

The standards that we set up in our lives need to be personal. I am not suggesting that we have a morality police set up a universal standard for the entire world; however I am suggesting that you know thyself and the things that are not healthy for you personally. Why do you continue to watch those things? You know the things that "haunt" your mind long after you are done watching them. Why do you still go back for more? You know the way you look at people around you in a demeaning way after you view those movies. Why do you continue to allow sewage into the fresh springs of your mind?

HOW WE SEE THE WORLD

There have been many studies done in recent years that link television watching and the effect that it has on the human mind with a person's overall behavior. They have researched everything from babies to the elderly and have seen how television consumption has helped to form the way individuals think, act and live; in some ways, very positively: Shows like "Sesame Street" and "Blue's Clues" have helped to begin develop children's mental development at very early ages. However, there are many others that have helped to cultivate a culture of violence, sexual promiscuity and disrespect that has reshaped the way that many people live.

Truly, it comes down to a very basic biological principle that we can see taking shape in many lives today. This master law taking place can be understood as "Like Begets Like". What this means at a very basic level in the biological world is that the offspring of a certain creature will resemble its parents. However, I want to tell you that in your life, **like will beget like**. In other words, you will find a transformation and a change happening internally based on what you are allowing to enter into the front doors of your life.

Scientifically, this has been proven in many different studies over the years. Concerning media violence, a well known follow up to a longitudinal study was done following a study which began in 1977 with children aged 6–10. The study, done by a group of doctors from the University of Michigan, [1] showed that over the course of 15 years, those who were watching more violent television at a young age were more violent with their spouses, committed more criminal acts, and had been convicted of crimes at a rate three times of those who weren't watching violent television. This is one of many studies that are out there that look at the effects of a person's life based on what they are letting in through their eyes.

It is no wonder that those who have started viewing pornography at a young age are more likely to be rapists or child molesters [2] or that playing violent video games increases the probability that you will be a violent person.[3] What we let in the doors of our eyes will begin to shape and change who we are.

Now, maybe you aren't watching porn or every new "hack 'em up" scary movie that enters into your local theatre, but I want you to think about the things that you *are* letting through that front door of your life. How are the things that you are letting into your life affecting you? Are you feeding a fear in your life by what you are watching on television? Are you massaging your personal insecurities by watching the perfect lives of TV families and comparing them to your own? Are you tickling your sexual desires by viewing things that get your heart racing and begin to tease you? Whatever it is, you are not alone.

Television, in itself, has become a staple in every home across America and in many parts of the world. I remember walking through the slums of Brazil and seeing monstrous satellite dishes on top of plywood shacks. Television is a mandatory essential in most homes today.

> "If everyone demanded peace instead of another television set, then there'd be peace."
>
> —**John Lennon** *(20th century British singer)*

In the US, TV watching is at an all time high. In 2009, a Neilson study came out showing that the average American is consuming 153 hours of television in their home each month.⁽³⁾ This works out to an average of over 5 hours of television every day of the year. This is more hours than many part time employees put in at their jobs. That, in itself, is reason to pay attention to your TV consumption. Imagine what you could do for yourself… your bank account… or the world in general if you were to focus five hours a day to a cause. Imagine what you could learn, create and share.

Then, there is the physiological effect that television watching has on you. As you are taking in your favorite sitcom, there are some interesting neurological changes taking place. Your brain actively switches from the left side (responsible for all of your logical thought and critical analysis) to your right. This is important because the right side of your brain isn't known for its critical analysis, but operates more at an emotional state and releases endorphins into your body which are natural sedatives. These endorphins being released can actually cause an **addiction to television consumption**. So, all those things that your mom said growing up were true! TV can actually make you dumber. (5)

So, let's take a look at our lives. What are the things that we are letting into our eyes… and ultimately our lives? What are the things that are entering in through the front door? How much time are we dedicating to those things that are sabotaging us and taking us further away from our goals? What are we going to do about it?

Let's look specifically at our TV consumption. I want you look at this and take an honest account of how much TV you are taking in on a daily basis. Your first desire will be to underestimate… so let's do an exercise.

From Monday to Monday, I want you to track your TV and online video and DVD and DVR consumption. Basically, if you are watching something on a screen, I want you to track it throughout your days. You will probably have different start and finish times on the same day and that is fine. Our goal is to find our total consumption. So, if you watch 2 hours of TV in the morning, 1 hour of YouTube in the afternoon and 4.25 hours of sitcoms at night, then your total consumption would be 7.25 for the day. Record your totals for the week and ask yourself how you feel about it.

Monday: _____

Tuesday: _____

Wednesday: _____

Thursday: _____

Friday: _____

Saturday: _____

Sunday: _____

Now, let's answer some questions about this exercise:

How do I feel about this week's TV consumption? Does it reflect a normal week for me?

_____
_____
_____
_____
_____
_____
_____
_____

For some, TV may be a very minimal part of your lives and I think that's great. However, for many of us, it is important that we get this one area under control for the betterment of humanity. Do you really want to invest 40 hours a week on watching a box or a screen on a wall? Do you really want to have a life where you are simply being spoon-fed someone else's ideas and creativity? Well, it's time to do something about it.

I want you to make a declaration of what the next 30 days of TV consumption is going to look like in your life. Maybe you want to do a total TV fast. Unplug it and put it in your closet for a month. Check out what you will be able to get done and the money that you will be able to save from a cable bill. Maybe it is simply cutting down TV consumption to one hour a day.

Whatever it is, truly challenge yourself. Your life is worth this change.

OK. Now let's take it to another level. There are other things in your life that you want to get rid of. There are other things that are entering into the doorway of our lives that need to be dealt with. As you have been reading this chapter, different things have come into the light. Maybe it's the websites you're visiting or the things you're reading or _____ (fill in the blank).

I want you to pick one more area of your life to address. You are going to answer three questions. Go ahead and write your answers below:

What area of my life do I want to work on?

_____
_____

How is it affecting me negatively?

_____
_____
_____
_____
_____
_____
_____
_____

What am I going to do about it? What is going to change?

_____
_____
_____
_____
_____
_____
_____
_____
_____
_____

By identifying those things that may have a negative effect on your life, you are empowering yourself to make positive changes. The first step in any major life transformation is the identification and implementation of new action. Take that goal that you have just set and begin down the road of implementation.

HOW THE WORLD SEES YOU

But what about the external effects that your eyes are making on your life that you may not even be aware of? Your eyes are communicating to the masses very important messages about you: They are telling the world to trust you or to look at you with unease. They are communicating your intentions. They are reflecting the "real you" to the world in which you live. No matter how hard you try to hide it, your eyes will not lie. So, we need to become aware of the message that our eyes are sharing with the world and work to improve that message.

Begin to pay attention to your next few conversations. Ask yourself, **"Are they looking me in my eyes?"** By putting your attention on their actions, you will subconsciously begin to pay a greater attention on your own eyes and what you are doing. How often do you look away? When you look someone directly in their eyes, how does that make you feel?

When you look someone in their eyes, you are sending a very strong message to them. You are letting them know that you are interested in what they are saying and, ultimately, in them as a person. You are communicating a sense of respect and letting them know that what they are saying is important to you. By keeping eye contact you are telling them that you really care about them and this simple fact could be the difference between a friend or an enemy… a client or another dead end… a romantic interest or another cold shoulder.

The great news is that if you are struggling with healthy eye contact, there are very simple steps that you can take to improve your eye contact with others. **Begin to cultivate some of these skills and watch your eye contact dramatically improve:**

1. Start with a group. Begin to work on your eye contact skills in the midst of a group conversation. Find the person that is speaking with your eyes and hold their eyes in your glance. Hold it long enough that you don't resemble a deranged lunatic and then look away. When you speak, look from person to person and hold the attention of the group.

2. One to one with the Bermuda Triangle. If you have been struggling with keeping eye contact, then this may make the endeavor so much easier. Try implementing what I like to call the "Bermuda Triangle". You will focus on the left eye of the person who is speaking to you for about ten to fifteen seconds. Then, move over to their right eye and then finally their mouth. This awareness of action will allow you to stay focused on the task at hand.

3. Listen with your eyes. A major part of communication is listening to another and this auditory action can be done with your eyes. As they are speaking and giving their ideas, pretend that you are listening with your eyes. You need to look at them to hear what they are saying. Examine their facial motions to gain a better perspective on what they are saying. Make mental notes of what you believe their inner motives or attitudes are about that subject based on your observations.

4. Woo someone with your eyes. As you begin to master this eye communication, you can reach the point where you attempt to communicate solely with your eyes. I recommend not using this technique on strangers, though some of you may try this on every person you meet at the bus stop. I will not be held responsible for the results, but try to woo someone with only your eyes. Look at them gently and let your eyes smile at them. Call them into your presence with your eyes and let them know that you want to know them by simply looking in their direction. The eyes have the ability to communicate very clearly... we just need to practice using them as a communication tool.

Out of the four action steps above, which one am I going to employ today?

_____

_____

After you do it, answer these questions:

How did it make me feel?

How do I think it was received by the person I was communicating with?

What advice would I give myself for the next time?

HOW WE SEE THE FUTURE

One final way to use your eyes to communicate a strong message is to allow yourself to use your eyes to see the future. The world is in desperate need of visionaries and people who will have a clear and inspiring vision of the coming days. They need you to be that person who has the ability to see the potential in themselves, others and ultimately the world.

In order to do this you have to be willing to see past your current circumstances or situations to the place that you want or need to be. You have to be willing to exit any comfort zone that you currently find yourself in and embrace a future that only lies in the vision of your mind's eye.

There is an ancient picture that is very well known in the United States today. It has a triangle with an eye in it and rays that seem to be shooting out in every direction. It can be found on US currency and it is known as "The All Seeing Eye of God" or "The Eye of Providence". This picture can be traced all the way back to Egyptian mythology and has even been linked to Freemasonry. However, I think the idea of an "all seeing" eye is quite interesting for us to imagine in our lives today.

Imagine if you could come to the place in your life where everything was about today. You would be able to set aside all the things of your past and focus solely on what was taking place today. Now, what if you were able to have a firm and balanced belief in your heart that there was a great plan for your life and that today was the first day in that plan coming to pass in your life? What if there was this vision that was birthed from inside of you that the tomorrows of your life were only going to become progressively better as you fulfilled the plans for your life? What if everything had the power to change and improve? What would change in your life?

With these thoughts in mind, I want you to entertain me for a minute. No matter what your thoughts were as we entered into this chapter, I want you to simply sit back and imagine with me. I want you to just think about what could possibly be. Take a moment to answer these questions:

If I knew that I could succeed, what would I reach for today? What would I attempt?

_____
_____
_____
_____
_____
_____

If I believed that there was a master plan for my life, what would my life look like according to the passions that I have in my heart?

_____
_____
_____
_____
_____
_____
_____
_____
_____

Setting all else aside, where would I like to see my life headed?

_____
_____
_____
_____
_____
_____
_____
_____
_____
_____

You see, when we talk about our eyes and the vision for our life, it encompasses so many different areas. There are things that we let in that end up affecting the interior of our lives, while there are things that end up coming out through the eyes that hinder our growth and progression in relationships, jobs and many different areas of our lives. And ultimately, our vision—or lack thereof—can cause the greatest damage by not allowing us to have any future at all… at least not the future that we deserve.

9

The Arm Pit: Controlling the Negative Odors of Life

A good friend recently sent me a commercial to watch on my Facebook page. It starts out in a locker room with a guy wearing only a towel and holding only a basketball. He pops his leg up on a bench, looks dead into the camera and says these simple words, **"I used to think that it didn't matter what deodorant I chose."** (awkward pause) Then with squinted eyes and a furrowed brow you heard one word, **"Dumb"**. This was followed by ten of the most uncomfortable moments of my life as he simply stared deeply into the camera and ultimately into my soul.

The commercial was ridiculous and that is why it became such a hit in the viral world; however the words were so true. It is dumb not to care about what we are using to negate the funk in our lives. This odor, or lack thereof, could mean the difference between getting a promotion or making a new friend or scoring that date with the girl of your dreams or getting the label of "that stinky guy" at work. And that odor needs to be controlled.

There is another odor that many of us don't think of as important that I would say is of equal, if not greater, importance. It is the putrid odor of the negative influences that we are allowing to enter into our lives and eventually take up root. These influences have many different forms and can be found in the newscasts we watch, the webpages we browse, the porn we ingest, the Gossip Magazines that fill our time in the lines of Walmart and many, many other areas that clog up our minds and lives. There are examples everywhere we turn and negativity can be found lurking around every corner.

Negativity is not something that discriminates. It doesn't matter your sex or race or age, there are a thousand negative stories that are directed specifically toward you. Whether it is the end of the world or the end of social security; the end of the economy or the end of your favorite TV show, there is plenty of negative stuff for you to focus your time and energy on. In our lives, we need to begin to exert control over those things that are allowed to come into our lives.

Imagine yourself as an air traffic controller. Your mind is the air that you have control over… this is the flight space that you are responsible for. You are not responsible for anyone else's air space, but you have complete and total control over your own. Your responsibility as the controller is to give permission or revoke permission for things that enter into your airspace. Nothing is allowed in your airspace without your consent. You have total control of what comes in and what doesn't. You are the controller.

The airspace of our life is that gray matter that lives between our ears—our mind. We have great control over those things that we let enter in and have the power to allow or disallow. Everyday we give permission or revoke the flying rights of many different situations and ideas that are floating all around us.

For the most part, we control everything, but there may be times when things sneak into our airspace. They didn't ask for express permission and they just showed up. Well, in that case, we have total authority whether or not we are going to let them land. As quick as they came in, we have the power to tell them to leave and get out. Nothing is allowed to land, or take root, unless we let it happen.

With this analogy in mind, let's take a look at some of the negative things that are fighting for the air space of our lives.

Perversion: There is an overwhelming desire in our sensual culture for perversion to enter into our lives, minds and airspace. There is nothing wrong with a beautiful woman or a handsome man. There is nothing wrong with someone taking notice of how ravishing someone is. The problem happens when that second glance turns into a lustful thought and your intentions turn carnal and reprobate.

Perversion, at its root, simply means twisted or misconstrued. It is taking something that is meant for good, and twisting it and turning it into something that it wasn't designed for. Pornography, for example, can be seen by some to be completely harmless and lacking of any true lasting damage to an individual. But, any person can easily see that the message of porn is very clear. Even if you're not into the darker side of porn, the message coming across in basic pornography to men about women is wrong. Some of the obvious conclusions can be seen from even the most "tame" porn:

Women are less than human. Whether it is Playboy calling them "bunnies" or Penthouse calling them "pets", porn oftentimes alludes that women are less than human and just here to service men. On the contrary, women have a great worth and they deserve to be treated with the utmost love and respect.

A woman's value rests in her attractiveness. The longer the legs and the more voluptuous the lips, the more worth that a woman has. This couldn't be further from the truth. A woman's value should never rest in her ability to arouse a man from her exterior, but who she really is as a person. A woman's value consists of all of her facets and not simply her curves and skin.

Women are a sport. "It is all about the game" or "She's just another notch in the belt" are thoughts that can come from viewing the pursuit of women as a sport. Guys say that they "won her over" or that they "scored last night". All of these sayings link women back to simply being another game for a guy to win. Porn is often about a man's ability to conquer or win the ultimate prize—sex with a beautiful woman.

Women are property. We've all seen the woman in a bathing suit lying on the sports car sending us the message that these two things come together. If you just buy that car, then you will have a greater chance of owning that woman too. Women are not the property of anyone. Porn often gives the picture that women are the property of man and they are to do whatever that man wants them to do.

"How do I know pornography depraves and corrupts? It depraves and corrupts me."

—**Malcolm Muggeridge** *(20th century English journalist and author)*

And these are pretty tame compared to a lot of the pornography coming out today. I am not even talking about the reality that women don't want to be raped... which is a form of porn now... or that underage girls shouldn't have sex... which is being portrayed in computer generated or animated porn... or that taboo sex is a valid choice... which gets millions of hits online each day. Through the consistent ingestion of these things, our views on women and sexuality begin to become perverted, or twisted, and become a disgusting aroma in our lives. We can't let the airplanes of perversion into our airspace.

Negative News: The University of Missouri researchers decided to examine why people were more attracted to the negative news that was being pumped through the air waves each and every day. Hooking the people up to monitors, they began to show them different news stories and they recorded the responses that they got from the participants. The researchers found that when they showed a local health threat, the participants showed a direct effect and their attention and memory both increased with the implementation of negative news. [1]

This shows us why this battle is so hard in a lot of our lives. Why do we find ourselves pulled to sit in front of the news station whenever there is some sort of calamity in the world? There is a physiological response that happens whenever we come face to face with negative news. There is a pull to take more in. We need another hit of what they have to give.

This influx of negative news begins to affect how we view the world. We begin to see everything through the eyes of this negativity. We begin to view the world as a dangerous place because there was a murder on the news. We begin to question our school system because a teacher had sex with a student. We begin to lose hope in our government because there was another illicit affair. Our complete world view begins to be torn down by the negativity that we are allowing in our lives.

We take the stories at face value and don't really look at them for what they are. We don't take into consideration that the murder was one person out of the city population of 100,000. This would mean that the percentage of you being that person who was murdered is .00001%. According to the National Highway Traffic Safety Administration, in 2009, per 100,000 populations, 11.01 people died. [3] This is a percentage of .00011%. Your chances of being killed in your Volvo far outweigh being gunned down by some creep. However, we fear the killer over the car. The news is affecting us.

What many people don't realize however is that negative news will follow them throughout the day. It becomes an active part of their thoughts and their conversation. Now, they are taking that negative thing that has become planted in them and planting it throughout their family and their workplace and becoming the Johnny Appleseed of negativity. There is an intense and overwhelming sensation to share bad news. We want other people to know about the bad stuff that we just became aware of.

The reality is that most things that we see in the media, we have absolutely no power in and of ourselves to change. We can't do anything about it, yet we are letting it come into our minds and steal away that sense of peace and joy that we should have each day. We need to take control over this medium and filter what is taking up residence on the landing strip of our cerebrum.

Gossip: Whether it is in magazines or in the company break room, gossip is a powerfully destructive force that has the potential to tear down and destroy. Yet, it is so attractive and tasty to the mental palette. We want to hear about the starlet's recent drug addiction or the coworker's affair. These things tickle our ears and promise to satisfy us in some weird way.

It is nothing new, however. Gossip has driven television and radio for decades and the kitchen table conversation for eons. It is all around us. The internet makes it so quick and easy to find. We can know someone's dirt within hours… or sometimes even minutes. We can follow it moment by moment and take that information and feed it to friends and family through blog posts or status updates. We can help perpetuate the gossip train.

What we often don't see is the damage that is caused by gossip. There is an ancient proverb that says, **"A troublemaker plants seeds of strife; gossip separates the best of friends."** (2) We find that the end goal of gossip is simply separation. Not always a separation that is physical, but this could happen with people choosing no longer to be friends because of gossip, but what I see more than not is an emotional separation from people and an erosion of trust. This erosion of trust begins to wear away at the very fabric of relationships and friendships. It tears away at the very fabric of society.

Just think back to a time in your life when you found out that people were talking about you. Maybe it was on the schoolyard or at a family reunion. Maybe what they were saying was true or a bold faced lie. How did it make you feel? Recalling the emotions that we experience during certain situations can help to control our actions toward others. If I remember how hurt and betrayed I felt because of someone gossiping about me, then I will be less apt to gossip about another.

"Some say that our national pastime is baseball. Not me. It's gossip."

—**Erma Bombeck** *(20th century US humorist)*

The best way to control the gossip that is coming from your lips is to control that which is coming into your ears. If we can begin to control our input, then we are sure to have a greater control on our output. Where are some hot beds of gossip for you? Whether it's the break room table or the afternoon phone calls to your best friend, begin to nix the gossip that you are allowing into your life and you will find a direct correlation to what is coming out.

Now I want you to write down a negative thing that is fighting for the airspace in your life. We all have different things that we struggle with and I want you to write down one thing from your life and then give me a little description of how you view that thing affecting you negatively:

REGAINING CONTROL OF THE SKIES

So now that we've identified a negative thing that could be trying to invade our airspace, let's look at some practical ways that we can regain control of the skies of our life. **How can we regain order and control?**

Our first step is to begin to control the flight patterns of our lives. When we begin to notice that there are things that are making their way into our lives, we need to reroute those things in other directions. For example, if we find ourselves being pulled into negative gossip in the break room, then we need to make a decision that we are not going to allow this to come into our lives anymore. We may make a statement and ask these individuals to refrain from the gossip. If you have built a good rapport with them, it may open up a very healthy discussion and cause some of the others to examine their air spaces. But if you don't have the rapport to do this, you may just need to go somewhere else. You may want to eat outside, find another place to take your break or just spend your lunch break taking a walk and partaking in some quality alone time.

Or, maybe you are struggling with porn and you desperately want to reroute the flight patterns to rid your life of this behavior. You may have reached the point where you feel powerless because of the habits that you have been forming over the last few years of your life. A great way to begin controlling the airways of your life is to employ the help of a friend.

There are some great programs out there that will help you by keeping track of the websites you visit and then notifying a friend if you begin to venture into unsavory waters. A great organization helping people break free from the grip of pornography is Covenant Eyes at **covenanteyes.com**. They offer an incredibly affordable program that is helping people all over the world by offering accountability and internet filter systems. There is another program that you can actually get for free called X3Watch which can be downloaded at their website at **x3watch.com**. This program is not only good for your computers, but can also be downloaded on to your smartphones and offer protection for the 21st century. Don't forget, you are the controller. If you want a change, you have to be the one to take the first step.

What about that negative thing that you wrote about? What are some practical things that you can actively do to bring about a greater control and change in that area? Write down a couple ideas here about what you can do.

_____
_____
_____
_____
_____
_____
_____
_____
_____
_____
_____

Another important thing to do in our lives is to begin to employ some healthy alternatives to those negative things that are currently taking up all of our time and energy. For every behavior that you want to change in your life, there are at least ten healthy alternatives to it. Your job is to identify what those things are. What do you want to see happen in your life and what things could fill your time and lead you in that direction?

What could you do with all the time that you've been wasting while you ingest negative news into your life? What could you do with the hours spent flipping from webpage to webpage? What would you be able to accomplish if you removed yourself from the TV for simply one hour a day? If you devoted only one hour a day to following the passions in your life, can you imagine what you could get done in a year?

THE BEST: A Life Manifesto

Imagine 365 hours of your life devoted to one thing. How many pages could you write? How many miles could you walk? How many songs could you create? How many conversations could you have? With only one hour a day.

And as this change begins to transform you, begin to share your story with others. I believe that the greatest asset that anyone has is their story. It has the power to inspire and direct others. There are many people in your sphere of influence right now that need you to lead them in the right direction. Maybe this is the first time that you are beginning to address different areas in your life and you are starting to sense some momentum toward a better future. As you implement these steps of change, you need to let your voice be heard and begin to help others.

There are many people in this world that need to begin controlling their airspace. For too long they have let anything and everything that wanted to enter in… in. And now their lives look like a cluttered junkyard with broken down cars and smashed up bath tubs. It is filled with rubble and the stench of decay and they wonder why their lives aren't moving in the direction that they want them to go. They need to clean out the junk and not let anything else in that they don't want to be there. They need to begin to control the boundaries of their life.

There is an often quoted study about boundaries and the fences we construct in our lives and it had to do with school children. It is said that during the early days of the progressive-education movement, an enthusiastic theorist decided that it would be wise to dismantle a chain link fence which surrounded a nursery-school yard. The idea was that the children would be able to have a greater sense of freedom with the fence removed and would no longer have any visible barrier to hold them back.

The fence was dismantled and the results were quite eye opening.

The children who were thought to attain a greater freedom ended up huddled together near the center of the playground. They didn't even venture near the edges of the playground but stayed close together in the security of one another. The lack of a fence limited the full expression and enjoyment of these children. The fence actually brought a greater sense of freedom to the children.

It is the same with us today. If we don't take an active role in defining those things that are allowed and aren't allowed in our lives... if we don't protect the fences in our lives... if we don't control the airspace of our minds... then we will often find ourselves huddled in the middle of our playground, not venturing to the edges of our potential. By disposing of the negative odors of our lives and building a strong boundary around the skies of our lives, we will ensure THE BEST life and a much more fulfilled existence.

10

The Brawn: 21 Days to "Pump You Up!"

The testosterone was so high that you could breathe it in like humidity. Muscles stacked on muscles were covered with extra small T-shirts while women gasped and men felt inferior. The contestants moved back and forth on the stage with hairless bodies shining brightly from copious amounts of oil. They were chiseled warriors… battling themselves for greater bulk and a more defined physique.

The champion arose from amongst the crowd, the third of three contestants who were about to do their final showdown. With mountains of muscles they flexed and showed their wares to the world. From biceps bulging to thigh muscles popping, these monstrous men moved in ways to accentuate their most valuable assets. At last, the decision was made. Third place went to Lou Ferrigno, the future Incredible Hulk, and the second place spot went to a Frenchman named Serge Nubret. And the winner of the 1975 Mr. Olympia went to none other than Mr. Arnold Schwarzenegger… winning the contest for the sixth year in a row and living up to his promise of "I'll be back".

I can honestly tell you that this chapter is not going to give you the tools that you need to become the next Mr. Olympia or to gain the chiseled physique of the Incredible Hulk or the Terminator. However, we are going to examine how important our muscle tone and development is to our lives. Then, we are going to take some simple steps to maintain and cultivate a healthy muscle growth in our bodies.

One thing that all of us are doing right now is getting older and it is the one constant that none of us can deny. With every breath we take and every second that passes, we are getting older and older. This aging process is affecting us, even if it is totally unbeknownst to our natural minds. There is a natural degradation and deterioration that is reshaping us in major ways. And one specific area that is under attack is our muscle.

Muscles are the strength and the power of your life and the tissues that serve as the power center of our bodies. Your body has three major muscle types:

Cardiac muscle, which keeps your heart pumping out that life juice, is responsible for keeping you alive.

Smooth muscle, which lines your arteries and bowels, keeps you regular.

Skeletal muscle, also known as lean muscle, is responsible for motion and movement and the external areas of the body.

For the sake of this chapter, we are going to focus on that skeletal muscle of our bodies.

Time brings on a natural deterioration to our skeletal muscles and these changes can begin to happen as early as thirty, but often can be seen more vividly around the ages of 40 or 50. It is simply your body obeying the old age adage of **"If you don't use it you lose it."** This becomes really easy to see with sagging skin, skinny arms and a waning muscle mass.

Many scientific studies have been conducted to prove this muscle loss. A recent study has shown that the total muscle mass that an individual has will normally decrease by nearly 50% between the ages of 20 and 90. This means that the muscle, or lack thereof, that you have at 20 will be double that which you will have at the ripe old age of 90. Statistically, you will lose 30% of your strength between ages 50 and 70 and another 30% of what's left will disappear each decade after that (1).

The great news for us, however, is that these are only statistics and you are someone who is not willing to accept someone else's statistics about your life. You have a desire to prove these negative statistics wrong and become stronger in the next decade than you are right now. You want to be healthier next year than you are right now and you want to get continually better with each passing breath. And the best news of all is that you can achieve this because you have the power to start today. No matter where you are starting from… it is never too late.

"There is an immeasurable difference between late and too late."

—Og Mandino *(20th century American author)*

I am reminded of a woman by the name of Ernestine Shepherd who was 56 years old and unhappy with her health.

She was ashamed at how she had let herself go and decided to do something about it, so she started to work out. She was 74 years old when I saw her on "Good Morning America" and at that time she had won... yes, I said "won"... 8 marathons! In addition to this, she ran 80 miles each week, bench pressed 150 pounds, did bicep curls with 15–20 pound dumbbells and was in the Guinness Book of World Records as the oldest female body builder.[2] Here was a woman who said "enough is enough" and got busy making her life what she wanted it to be. Let us draw inspiration and declare that it is *never* too late and today is the day!

The first thing that I want you to know is that no matter where you currently are, today is the starting place and the **best place** for you to begin. I need you to wash away any disappointment or regret about how you got to this place. Regret is never going to transform into the motivation that you need to get where you want to go. You need inspiration and a burning desire in your heart for a better future. This, and only this, will get you moving in the right direction. So let's start there.

Why do you want to develop muscle? What is your motivation? Is it so the "big kids" won't kick sand in your face at the beach? Is it so that "smoking hot" coworker will notice you? Is it so you can spend hours in front of the mirror flexing and telling yourself how beautiful you are? Well, these things may motivate you for awhile, but in the long run they are going to wear off. You'll beat up the kid at the beach, the smoking hot chick will hook up with your boss in an attempt to climb the corporate ladder, and you will grow tired of counting the muscle dimples on your butt cheeks and that motivation will be gone. **(Thank God!)** You need to begin to find something that will provide you great motivation over a long period of time. Let's look at a few motivating factors that will last for the long haul:

I want my kids to see my lifestyle and be inspired to take a proactive role in the health of their lives.

Use your children as a motivating factor for your acquisition of muscle mass. When you are working out, think about the inspiration that you are being to them. Think about how they are looking at your life and the inspiration that you can give them to live a healthier life.

> "To bring up a child in the way he should go, travel that way yourself once in a while."

—**Josh Billings** *(pen name of 19th century humorist writer)*

I never want my health to stop me from doing what I want to do.

Begin preparing today for all of the amazing things that you want to do tomorrow. If someone gave you an all expense paid trip to hike the Himalayas, would your lack of leg muscles force you to tell this person that you'll have to pass on a once in a lifetime experience? If your husband offered to take you on a backpacking trip across Europe would you have to tell him "no" because you couldn't carry a backpack? Commit to be proactive today about the future you want to have tomorrow.

I don't want to end up like my parents.

I normally wouldn't take a negative stand to inspire. "I don't want…", in this situation however, has provided me with an extremely motivating force. My mother died in her early 50's from a heart attack and I have taken this personal genetic reality and used it as an inspiration to work out and stay healthy. Maybe your parents struggle with muscle loss, obesity or weak bone structure. Take that negative and use it as a positive in your life.

I want to beat the odds.

For some of you rebels out there, you're going to love this one: Get an attitude that you simply don't want to be like everyone else. You aren't going to lose muscle mass just because everyone else does. You aren't going to get weaker as you age, but you are going to get stronger. You are going to beat the odds and the statistics and show them that you aren't a follower, but a leader and an inspiration to many. This is a great way to express rebellion! Rebel against the status quo!

So now I want you to write out three motivating factors that will help you focus on your muscle development. I don't want you to simply write "To beat the odds," I want to know why. What odds do you want to beat? Why do you want to beat those odds? What does that mean to you? What would completion of this goal mean to you? What difference will it make to your life?

OK, here you go. I want three motivating factors for muscle development. Go!

1._____
_____
_____
_____

2. _____
_____
_____
_____

3. _____
_____
_____
_____

Now that we've written down some motivating factors, I want you to find a visual representation of what you would like to see developed in your body. What would your perfect body structure look like? Some may be going for the Mr. Universe look but others would be happy with Vin Diesel or Ben Affleck. Ladies, maybe it is a Jennifer Lopez, Queen Latifah or Katie Holmes. Find someone that inspires you and print out their picture and keep it close to you.

Now that you've defined the "why" behind the "what", let's put the "drive" behind the "butt". We are going to look through your major muscle groups. We will be looking at four things—the major muscle group, the location of that muscle group, an exercise that will strengthen that muscle group and a sample stretch to do before and after you work out that muscle group. Stretching is very important and you should stretch before and after each exercise. This is by no means an exhaustive list, but simply something to get you thinking. Begin to examine this chart and put a star next to the muscle groups that you'd like to focus on for the next couple of weeks: [3]

Major Muscle Group	Location	Exercise to Strengthen	Sample Stretch
Abdominal	Stomach	Crunches and Leg Raises	Not commonly stretched before or after exercise
Gluteus	Buttocks	Squat and Leg Press	Sit on chair, cross leg over thigh of bent leg, lean forwards.
Biceps	Front of Upper Arm	Bicep Curls	Sit down on the floor and put your palms down behind you with fingers facing away from you. Walk your hips away from your hands
Triceps	Back of Upper Arm	Push Ups, Tricep Extensions and Dips	Put both hands over your head and bend one at the elbow so that it's "scratching your back". Take the other hand and lightly push at the elbow.
Quadriceps	The front of your thigh	Squats, Lunges, Leg Press, Stair Climbing	While standing, bend at knee and bring leg back. Grab ankle with hand and lightly pull while pushing knees together.
Gastrocnemius & Soleus	Back of the lower leg	Calf Raises, standing or sitting	Lunges with a straight back leg for gastrocnemius. Lunges with bent knees for soleus.

Major Muscle Group	Location	Exercise to Strengthen	Sample Stretch
Hamstrings	The back of your thigh	Squats, Lunges, Leg Extensions, and Leg Curls	While standing, place the heel of the leg to be stretched on a chair with the leg straight. Bend over at the waist while pulling your toes back to your body.
Deltoids	Top of the shoulders	Push Ups, Bench Press, side and rear Arm Raises	Put both hands over your head and bend one at the elbow so that it's "scratching your back". Take the other hand and lightly push at the elbow.
Erector Spinae	Lower back	Back Extensions	Kneel on all fours and round your back up.
Latissimus Dorsi & Rhomboids	The back: Lats are the large triangular muscles in the midback	Pull Ups, Chin Ups, or Lat Pull Downs	Lats: Put both hands over your head and bend one at the elbow so that it's "scratching your back". Take the other hand and lightly pull at the elbow.
	Rhomboids are the muscles between the shoulder blades	Chin Ups and Bent Arm Rows	Rhomboids—"hug yourself". Cross arms in front of yourself and put hands on shoulder blades.
Trapezius	Large muscles in upper- and mid-back	Upright Rows and Shoulder Shrugs	Upper trap stretch: Sit in a chair, put your left hand behind you. Tilt your head so your right ear moves toward your right shoulder. Repeat on the other side.

Major Muscle Group	Location	Exercise to Strengthen	Sample Stretch
Obliques	The side of the body	Twisting crunches and rotary torso	Lie on your back with your arms extended out ("T" shape). Bend both knees. Rotate your hips and put your bent legs on the floor on your side.
Pectoralis	Front of the upper chest	Push Ups, Pull Ups, and Bench Presses	Stand and hold both arms out at shoulder height with your palms forward. Pull your arms back

Now that you've gained a better understanding of the major muscle groups, we are going to pick a few different areas that we want to focus on. I believe in setting goals that are attainable and once those goals are reached, you will be propelled to make more goals and reach them. There have been proven studies that show that 21 days will turn an action into a habit, so I want us to pick six different muscle groups from these areas that we are willing to commit the next 21 days to. Go ahead and write the major muscle groups here:

1. _____
2. _____
3. _____
4. _____
5. _____
6. _____

Now I want you to take those six muscle groups and split them in half. So three will be in one group and three will be in another. It will be good to link these together like "upper body" and "lower body" or "arms" or "legs" or some other way that you like. It doesn't really matter how you split them, just in some way that will be easy for you to distinguish between the two. Put an "A" next to three of them and a "B" next to the other three.

Now you have an "A" workout and a "B" workout. Every day of the week you will be exercising three of your major muscle groups. One day you will do your "A" group and the next day you will do your "B" group. You can choose what exercises you want to do. Whether you choose to do one rep or ten doesn't really matter to me. Also, I don't care if you choose to do one exercise or five different ones that work that major muscle group. I just want you to begin doing something and for many of us, that **something** is a lot more than the **nothing** that we are currently doing.

"Get busy living or get busy dying."

—Andy Dufresne *(character in the movie "Shawshank Redemption")*

After we have developed our "A" and "B" workouts, we are going to commit to exercise these major muscle groups for the next 21 days. There is a great website that you can use in order to help you keep track of this 21 day transformation of your life. It is called **habitforge.com**. This website is designed to help people forge new and healthy habits in their lives. You can sign up for free and have access to work on one habit at a time. The website will send you out an email each day asking if you were successful reaching your goal the day before. If you answer 'yes', then you will move forward toward your 21 day goal. If you were not successful, then you will have to start over from scratch in your attempt to reach the 21 day goal. For a minimal cost, you can make as many goals as you want and keep track of them on the website, but for the sake of this exercise, you can join for free and simply make your goal:

"Did I exercise my muscles?"

You will be responsible for keeping track of which muscles you have to work out. Simply answer the email with a yes or a no (preferably a resounding **"yes!"**) and after you have completed this new habit for 21 straight days, you can reassess. Do you want to add more exercises or change the exercises up? Do you want to increase the number of reps or exercises that you are doing for a specific area? How do you want to see your goals evolve? After reaping the benefits of 21 days of exercise, I am sure that you are going to be energized and excited about the results that you are witnessing and the increased strength that you are experiencing.

For some of us, we may have trouble in the midst of the 21 days. We may find ourselves doing really well for the first few days, but then our motivation begins to wane and we find ourselves not being motivated to exercise. Those first few weeks are truly some of the hardest days so I want to give you a few tricks that I have used that have helped me stay motivated even when the going got tough:

Use music to motivate. I have used nothing with greater success than music. It, single-handedly, has motivated me to keep going and not give up and has pushed me to go on when all I wanted to do was quit.

When working with music and exercise, you have to pick music that has a message that will push you forward and a beat that will keep you going and something that you will enjoy listening to. Many friends of mine choose to listen to heavy metal which causes them to "dig deep". Personally, that would just give me a headache; I look for something with a strong beat (whether it is hip hop or techno) and a great message of not giving up or quitting. Check out the website, **thebestmanifesto.com** for some different playlists and some ideas from some other people.

Visual motivation. Take that photo that you printed out earlier of your "goal person" and put it where you can see it. Take a photo of yourself and the areas of your body that you aren't happy with and put it in your exercise area so that you can always see what you are leaving behind. Put up some motivating quotes in different key places that tell you to keep going. There are some great examples on the website, **thebestmanifesto.com**, for you to use.

Reward yourself. Set a goal and make a reward for yourself. For example, **"If I increase my bicep size by two inches… I will treat myself to a two hour massage."** Buy a gift certificate for the massage and keep it right by your weights. Every curl you do is getting you closer to that massage. Or, plan a vacation at the beach and purchase it with a stretch of time to redeem it (like a four month time period). As soon as you reach that goal on the bench press or a continuous number of pushups, you are allowed to redeem that vacation. If you don't reach the goal, then you don't redeem it. If you miss the redemption date, you can kiss the vacation goodbye. Do you want to talk about motivation? Losing money and a week at the beach is always a good motivating factor for me. The key is to buy it now and give yourself something to fight for.

PROTEIN—WHERE'S THE BEEF?

Another important ingredient in the recipe of brawn is the consumption of protein and its interactions with the muscles in our body. We need to assure that our diet is complementing the hard work that we are putting in day in and day out. For some of us, we are not sure how to measure our "muscle building foods" with all of the other things that we ingest. The information out there can be conflicting and confusing and we choose to simply keep sucking back Big Macs until we find something we can understand. Well, throw the Mac in the trash, because a protein revelation is about to take place.

There are many different thoughts about the proper diet for a healthy life, and I am not trying to tackle that subject in this book nor do I have the qualifications of a registered dietician or a PhD. I do, however, understand that there have been countless studies done on the effect of protein on muscle development, which places a high value on this subject when it comes to my continual development of strength.

Proteins are key to this muscle development and are part of every cell, tissue and organ in our bodies. Proteins are consistently being broken down and then replenished. The protein in the food that we eat ends up being digested into amino acids that are later used to replace the proteins that have been used through daily activities. We find protein in all kinds of different food that we ingest:

Meats, poultry, fish, eggs, seeds, nuts, tofu, legumes, milk, milk products, grains, some vegetables and some fruits.

In the last few decades, we have witnessed an incredible interest and development in dietary supplements that increase the protein that we take into our body. You can now buy protein bars, protein shakes, protein drinks and protein powders. You can find whey protein and soy protein and casein protein and some other varieties on the shelves of your local health store. Protein has taken an incredible turn as it is becoming one of the most popular key words in health and exercise.

But how much protein do you really need? Well, that is a common question and could be answered pretty easily using a simple math equation. According to the Food and Nutrition Board, the recommended daily allowance is 0.36 grams or protein for every pound that you weigh. So, if you weigh 200 pounds, the recommended daily allowance if 0.36 x 200 = 72 grams. This number is a very conservative number and if you are interested in truly developing your muscle mass; you will have to see that amount of protein increase.

I recommend that you get onto the website **HowMuchProtein.com**[1] for a complete personalized recommendation for your protein intake. It will allow you to choose between your overall goals of muscle building, endurance, weight loss or power and speed. I want you to have a personalized number so that you find that your goals are being completed. Once you decide on your goals, write your protein daily allowance here: _____

Now it is time to raid the pantry and begin learning about the amount of protein in your foods. If you have purchased your meat fresh, you may have to get online to discover the protein content. I want you to write down 10 items that you *think* have protein in them and write what you *think* their protein content is in grams. Then, grab the package out of the fridge or pantry and check out the actual protein content and write it below:

Food Item	I Thought it Had	It Really Has
1.		
2.		
3.		
4.		
5.		
6.		
7.		
8.		
9.		
10.		

This activity may have been shocking for a couple different reasons. First, we may have realized how clueless we are about the amount of protein in foods and under- or overestimated in big ways. Secondly, we may have discovered that foods that we thought were high in protein really weren't. This increased awareness of what we are ingesting will help us reach the goals that we are reaching for in muscle development. Our major goal is simply to wash away ignorance and to become an active participant and not simply a passive recipient of life.

Now, let's look back at our goal number and the foods that we just investigated. In order to reach that minimum goal, what would you have to eat? Let's make up three sample "menus" using the foods that we looked at to see how much we would have to eat to reach our protein goal in a 24 hour period of time. This will cause us to become aware of protein and its presence in the foods that you eat.

Sample Menu 1	Sample Menu 2	Sample Menu 3
_____	_____	_____
_____	_____	_____
_____	_____	_____
_____	_____	_____

I know that tackling these areas in your life can be very difficult and cause you to examine different areas that you may have been putting off for some time. It may have caused some tough memories to reemerge and may have even tempted you to just give up and move on to the next chapter or quit on the book altogether. But… you didn't. Things are changing in your life and you are willing to address areas that have been left untouched for years. There is a change in the air and you can feel it. You want to do something great with your life and are willing to put in the work to get where you want to be. With this sense of tenacity, there will be no stopping you!

Imagine if the world didn't end in 12 months. Imagine that you didn't die in some catastrophic cosmic accident. Imagine that you were still alive and breathing in one year's time. Where would you want to be physically? What would you want to look like? How would you want your life to be different? Because, if you are still around in 12 months, you are not going to be in that place if you don't start doing something about it. You are going to be in the exact same spot that you are today. Nothing would have changed and you are just going to be a few breaths closer to death. I don't think that is the life that you want to be living and the fact that you are still reading tells me that you desperately want something different from your life. You want your life to count. You want to make a difference. And I believe that you will.

Take a deep breath and start today. 21 days will make a habit so let today be day one. Get started and begin to watch your life change. You are the only one in control right now so become an active participant in the life that you are choosing to live. There is no time like the present… so, shut this book right now and let's get "pumped up"!

11

The Ears: Listening for Life

So I was watching a guy as he moved from person to person and group to group at a party I was at. He surely held the gold medal for working the room. He was a pro… a champ… an expert. He had the grace of a gazelle and the smile of a used car salesman. There was a rhythm to his talk and a gallop in his walk. He crept closer to my friend who was leaning hard against the wall and I just smiled at what I was about to witness.

You see, my friend is one of those honest types who tell you exactly how he is doing even when you don't really care and can't do anything to help him. He is a talker and loves to lay his life out there. He lets you know exactly what is wrong and leaves no details uncovered. I watched as the sweet talking stranger inched closer. I smiled because I love to watch uncomfortable moments unfold… especially when they don't involve me.

"Hey Buddy. My name's Robert. How are you doing tonight?"

"Well…" Long dramatic pause that my friend is well known for. "It's actually quite terrible for me right now. I just got laid off from my job and then I took this other position and they are messing around with my hours and my wife can't stand it and she's even questioning if she wants to stay married—" He still hadn't taken a breath. "—and if this thing doesn't work I don't know what I'd end up doing because I'd end up out on the streets or living back with my folks and they are getting too old to take care of me which just brings…" And he went on and on.

The "crowd worker" interrupted. "Listen, you have a great night tonight and I'll see you later." Then the guy was off to his next group with the same plastic smile and fake questions that made people think he cared. He really didn't want to be bothered by what my friend had to say. He really didn't care about how he was doing. He was only out for himself.

This story is repeated at thousands of dinner parties and church gatherings and little league games and family reunions. Plastic smiles that share lies about true interest… when the only expected response is the staple answer to "How are you doing?" and that is "Fine".

But if we truly want to reach the place where we are living a healthy existence while impacting the lives of others, we are going to have to reach a point where we have a firm understanding of the power of listening and employ it in our daily lives. If may be something that we have never addressed or honestly looked at. We may be mirroring the attitude of our parents when it came to listening to us, or carry the same tone as our boss who has a "My way or the highway" way of listening. It doesn't matter what we've seen or even what we've employed in our lives up to now. We can learn what it means to effectively listen and practice it each and every day.

LISTENING vs. HEARING

Many people fail to distinguish between listening to someone and hearing what someone is saying. However, these two things couldn't be further from one another. If we are going to improve our listening ability, then we need to take an honest look at what we are doing in our lives today and how it is perceived by others. Are we listening or simply hearing them?

Hearing: I like to describe hearing as a very passive act. We allow our ears to receive sound, but fail to pay attention to those things that are entering into our eardrums. We may gain some knowledge by what we are hearing, but it is at a very one-dimensional and at a static level.

Listening: I like to describe listening as a very active act. We are paying close attention to the sounds that enter into our ears. And then, when we hear them, we begin to take and apply thoughtful attention to them. We may find ourselves leaning forward in our seats and giving verbal clues that we are connecting with the message that is being given to us. The speaker can tell that we are engaged and we care.

As a communicator, I have seen the difference between these too many times. I share with a crowd and as I look out there are some who may be flipping through a brochure or fumbling with their cell phone, but then there are others who are leaning forward in their seats with their eyes heavy on me. They want to hear the next words that are going to come out of my mouth. They are connected in every way and are truly *listening* to the words that I am sharing.

And then, at the completion of my teaching, I will have some people shake my hand and walk out of the door appearing to be no different than they were when they came in while others will come and share about how influenced they were from the teaching and how their lives will never be the same. Now this is a statement that I have heard many times and I know that it is not because of anything that I did. If it was solely because of the quality of my message, then everyone's lives would be changed. Instead, only a portion of the crowd is forever changed and it is because they positioned themselves in a place to listen.

"When you are listening to somebody, completely attentively, then you are listening not only to the words, but also to the feeling of what it being conveyed, to the whole of it, not part of it."

—Jiddu Krishnamurti
(20th century Indian writer and philosopher)

Remember, listening is an *active* act. This means that we have the power to position ourselves in a place to hear. We have the power over whether we are listening or simply hearing something come at us. We have the ability to walk away after hearing "just another thing" being spoken to us—or have our worlds rocked and lives altered. So let's look at some keys to become an active listener:

Sit up, shut up and turn your phone off. Here you have three things that all tie together to assure that you are listening to the message that is coming forth. Sit up on the edge of your seat. If you do this, it forbids your body from becoming too comfortable and getting sleepy or disconnecting from what you need to hear. Don't talk to the people around you when there is something that you need to be listening to. Tell them that you will talk to them after you are done listening. Don't let someone else steal your ability to have your life changed. Finally, turn your phone off. There is nothing worse than being connected to a thought or an idea that is coming forth and feeling the vibration from your cell phone radiate up your leg. Let them leave a message and return the call after you are done listening.

Take notes and apply the senses. When you sit down with a pen and paper or a computer that is open to a blank text screen, you are sending a message that you are expecting to learn something that is so important that you don't ever want to forget it. There are even apps that you can use on your phone that assures that you are always ready to take some notes. A popular and **free** computer program out there is called "Evernote". It is available in nearly every platform that you would want and seamlessly passes your notes from your phone to your laptop to your PC. It has great search capabilities and did I mention that it was free? The more things that you can do to apply additional senses to a presentation, the greater ability you will have to be forever changed. Use your ears and your eyes and employ your hands as you type and write and nod your head and let a guttural sound escape from your larynx as you send positive feedback to the one communicating with you. It will pay off. I promise!

Fight back the Attila the Hun conquest tactics. Many reading this book right now are leaders. We see a problem and the first thing that we want to do is fix it. We may have "Type A" personalities and equate having to be quiet and listen to our upcoming proctology appointment… but it must be done. There are times when we need to solve the problem or pull the trigger or make the decision. But, when we talk about listening, sometimes we simply need to bite our tongues. This is where the computer or pad of paper will come in necessary. As you are listening and gain solutions in your mind's eye... write them down. This will allow you to give the solutions or ideas in the proper time and cause you not to hijack the time. In doing this, you are sending a strong message that what the person is saying is important to you and that you care about their opinions on the subject. Also, by allowing them to speak, we may be able to gain some insight which will cause our solutions to be much better than they would be without it.

"The ear of the leader must ring with the voices of the people."

—**Woodrow Wilson** *(28th President of the United States)*

Try to hear the emotion or "heart" behind the words. This one simple concept has improved my listening capabilities more than any other. When I sit down for a meeting or a "heart to heart" with a friend, I make a conscious effort to listen to the emotion behind the words that are being said. In other words, I try to take their words and look past them to see where they are coming from. **Why are they so passionate about a certain subject? Does this anger them or sadden them and how does that emotion affect how their ideas are coming across?** I'm sure that we have all been in a situation where someone's emotions have gotten the best of them and they were unable to complete the message that they were trying to get across. If we are able to understand where that emotion is coming from than we will have a greater understanding of their feelings and ideas.

Be empathetic and nonjudgmental. Empathy is a beautiful word which, if rightfully employed, has the ability change the world. Empathy simply means **"the ability to understand and share the feelings of another"**. To become an effective listener, there is no better way to send that message than to be an empathetic listener. You are trying to understand the person's feelings and where they are coming from. You want to know why they feel as passionately as they do about a certain subject and then to allow yourself to feel a little bit of what they feel. Try to listen in a place of nonjudgmental thought, listening to their entire message before you pass judgment on it. This will allow you to communicate from an educated position versus simply giving your predisposed idea on a certain subject.

Know when to quit listening and start talking. Communication is not simply about listening, but also giving feedback and personal opinions about a certain subject that is covered. When we reach the point where we understand the message that is coming forth and it is our turn to reciprocate, it is important that we allow ourselves to speak and help that conversation to grow. If we are in a classroom, we should be the ones asking questions as this is a part of active listening. We are sending a message to our instructor that we heard what they said and that we are processing it through discourse. Many instructors will embrace the conversation and it may even give you a few bonus points on that next essay question you are going to have to answer.

Now that we've looked at some very practical advice on how to improve your listening skills, I want you to pick three things that you are going to do to improve your listening skills in the next 90 days. You can take these

things from the list above or make your own. **The only rule is that you need to be committed to dedicating the next 21 days to developing these different skills.**

1. _____
   _____
   _____

2. _____
   _____
   _____

3. _____
   _____
   _____

Now that we are challenging ourselves to listen and not simply hear, let's look at the different groups that we need to be listening to.

OTHERS

This is probably the most well known and understood group that we need to employ strong listening skills with. We need to listen to what other people are saying and gain an incredible knowledge and wisdom from them. We need to be open to new thoughts and ideas and concepts that can often come from the most unlikely sources. The "others" are all around us and we need to pay close attention to them.

What message are the "others" in your life giving you right now? Are they challenging you to better yourself or encouraging you to just keep on keeping on? Are they propelling you forward in your career, family and social life or does it feel like they are secretly trying to sabotage you

THE BEST: A Life Manifesto

with the words that are coming out of their mouths? Do you feel smarter or stronger or better equipped for life from spending time with them or do you leave drained, disheartened and dumber? You need to be able to filter the people in your life and this filtering can be done with your ears.

When you hear an overwhelming amount of negativity and gossip and trash that you don't want to clog your life up with, allow your ears to filter those people out of your life. You may need to boldly tell them that you don't want to hear that stuff. But, sometimes, people are so conditioned to act like this that it will take a lot more than your chastisement to get them on the straight and narrow. In those situations, you may simply need to tell them "Adios" and keep moving. It may hurt for a moment, but in time you will soar with that dead weight cut from you.

On the other hand, you need to keep those who build you up close by. Those who are speaking life and hope into you need to be on your speed dial. Their words enter into your ears and water the garden of your existence, making you happy and healthy and longing for more out of life. You want to have a continual input from these individuals and try to reciprocate their impact on your life by speaking life into others in your day to day interactions.

Then there are the new connections that you have the potential to meet each and every day. Your ears need to be open and attentive to the opportunities that exist all around you. You will never get to the next level of your life with *only* the friends and acquaintances that you have today. You will have to make new relationships that will take you to the next level. People will come into your life who will want to stand with you and assist you getting to a greater place. But you will only find these people if you walk with a greater awareness. Perk your ears up and you may be surprised at the wonderful doors that open all around you.

YOURSELF

If I have said it once, I want to say it a million times: **"You have great advice for yourself!"** There is something dwelling on the inside of you that wants to lead you toward a better life and provide you with great insight over the best direction and choices for your life. The problem with most people isn't that this voice doesn't exist, but that we don't ever take the time to listen to that one person who knows you better than anyone… **you!**

You simply need to take time out of your busy life to listen to yourself. For some reason this is a very difficult concept to embrace in the western part of the world. We often think that physical inactivity equates with laziness, but this couldn't be further from the truth. We are only going to be able to operate at our greatest potential when we have a healthy inner dialogue going on and we are listening to ourselves.

This will only happen, however, when we make time for it to happen. Here are a couple ways to assure that you are giving yourself adequate time to listen to yourself:

Schedule It: If you don't schedule it, it probably won't happen. Put it into your schedule and even make it a repeating event. Every day at a certain time or Monday, Wednesday and Friday of each week will be a time for you to listen to yourself.

Start Small: Give yourself 10 minutes a day. Start small and allow it to grow from there. Many people are intimidated at being alone and quiet with themselves. You don't need to have this extended 12 hour session. Once you see the amazing effects from your time of listening to yourself, you will want that time period to grow exponentially.

Start Early or Late: Pick a time when your house is quiet and you can be still and listen without any distractions. There is no better time to do this than really early or really late. I personally prefer early because my brain is at its freshest point and not diluted by the issues of a full day. But, **know thyself** and choose accordingly. Just make sure it's quiet and distraction free.

Enter into your time with a question:
Start with a question that you're dealing with at the forefront of your mind. Search within for an answer to that question. Maybe your question has to do with your present job situation or a relationship that you are considering. Whatever it is, I want you to make sure that it is something that you really want wisdom about or an answer to.

Listen with a pencil, pen or keyboard:
Type that question across the top of a page and wrestle with the question in your mind, beginning to answer it in your own words. As fresh ideas enter into your mind, write them on the paper in front of you. Don't dwell on them or try to develop them. Just write them down in their roughest form and allow yourself to return to those ideas later.

Add one of your own. Remember the purpose is to take time for **YOU** to listen to **YOU**. What is one thing that you can implement in your personal life? Go ahead and write it down.

_____
_____
_____
_____

LIFE

I am a strong believer that our lives are great communicators but we are very poor listeners. Everything that happens in our lives, whether physically, emotionally, mentally or spiritually, is sending us a message about how we are living and what we are making from our lives. We need to become active listeners to the rhythms of our lives and begin to move in the healthy currents that surround us instead of fighting against the tide.

Potential, possibility and opportunity lie all around us. The only difference between those who are grabbing a hold of it and those who aren't is ambition and the ability to listen. **What are the messages that your life is sending you? What is the product from the decisions of your life and what are you doing to adjust to them? Are you listening?**

Your body is sending you a message today… are you listening? If you are overweight or underweight and tired all the time, a message is coming forth… are you listening? If you feel stressed out from the moment you rise till you pass out each night, a message is coming forth… are you listening? If you toss and turn every night and can't get a good night's sleep, a message is coming forth… are you listening?

What is the message that your body is giving you today? Take five minutes and really think about the question. If you were to listen to your body, what do you think the message is that is trying to get across?

_____
_____
_____
_____
_____
_____
_____
_____
_____
_____
_____
_____
_____
_____
_____
_____
_____
_____
_____
_____
_____
_____

_____
_____
_____
_____
_____
_____
_____
_____
_____

You have the power to do something about it. Flip over to the chapter on the heart or the brawn to gain some practical advice on how to address this message. Once your body begins speaking, we have to do something about it. If we don't, then it will just get louder and louder and harder and harder to dig out of it. The best thing to do is start today.

In addition to this inner dialogue that is taking place, there is also an external dialogue that life is having with you. All around you there are opportunities that life is opening the doors to. We will often simply walk right past these open doors because we are not listening to the message that life is trying to send us. In order to achieve THE BEST life possible, we need to begin to listen and walk through those open doors.

I have a simple prayer that I say in my life: **"Lord, open doors and shut doors and give me the courage to walk through the doors you open and not mourn the doors you close. Amen."** Since I started praying that prayer many years ago, I have seen many doors opened and even more slammed in my face. In the beginning, I was upset about the ones that shut, but hindsight always proved to show me how their closure was for my greater benefit. On the other hand, those that opened weren't always the ones that I expected to open, but I kept my word and have walked through every one of them. In the beginning it was difficult, but after receiving incredible benefits and blessings, I now sit in eager expectation for the next doors that are opened in my life. Even this very book, the words that you are currently reading, is a testament to the commitment to walk through open doors.

Now I want to ask you, **"What doors have been opening up in your life that you have been too fearful to walk toward?"** Maybe you have been too scared to walk through them until now. Maybe you understand the quote that says:

> ## "It's not the open doors that scare me; it's simply the dark hallways."
> ### —Unknown

The scary part isn't the actual opportunity, but not knowing what success or failure looks like. The unknown stops us from taking that first step which ultimately stops us from our destiny. The place that we need to reach is where we are listening to life and acting in a place absent of fear…. where we are taking those first steps in spite of the dark hallways.

What am I NOT striving for in my life because I am scared of the dark hallways?

_____
_____
_____
_____
_____

If the light were on in the dark hallways of my life, what would I strive for?

The lights in the dark hallways of life are connected to motion sensors and won't illuminate until they are triggered. You will often find that *after* you take the first steps into the dark hallways, the lights will all come on and you will be able to see clearly. However, most of us never witness this because we are left standing at the doorways looking at the darkness. I want to encourage you to step out in spite of the darkness and you will often find life getting a lot brighter as you do!

IT'S A JUNGLE OUT THERE

I think that we can learn a lot from our friends in the animal kingdom. There are animals throughout the world that rely almost completely on their sense of hearing for their safety, security and guarantee of food that will keep them alive.

Without their sense of hearing, they wouldn't survive. In many ways, our lives reflect this same reality.

Frogs are a great example of how listening can greatly affect your life. The male frog sends out a sound that actually consists of two parts. The first part is heard by the other male frogs and it warns of the presence of another male intruder while the second part is heard only by the female and informs them that there is a potential mate in the area. **It's amazing how a frog's croak one minute can reflect Michael Buffer, the famed referee in boxing and wrestling, saying "Let's Get Ready to Rumble!!!" and the next minute can reflect Marvin Gaye singing, "Let's Get it On".**

Or what about a mother elephant who can make great noises with her trunk, a sound which can be heard for a great distance in every direction, but when calling her calf, simply slaps her ears against her head and the calf comes running. This baby needs to make sure that he's listening to his mama.

In our lives, we need to be truly exercising the discipline of listening. It sends a strong message to others that we care. It builds our knowledge base and helps us grow as individuals and assures that we are consistently moving in the direction of growth, development and becoming the incredible creations that we were created to be!

12

The Soul: Spiritual Awakening

I once heard a story about a young, devout Buddhist monk who sat outside of the temple two thousand years ago. This monk would sit from before sunrise to long after sunset and repeat two words over and over again. Day after day he came back to the same spot and repeated those same words in a hope to acquire grace or a greater understanding of the spirit.

One day, his teacher came and sat across from him and began rubbing two bricks together. He sat and rubbed all day long as the student repeated his two words over and over again. Every now and then the student would crack his eye, look over at the teacher, catch himself peeking and return to his chant. After about six hours, he finally stopped chanting, opened his eyes and addressed his teacher.

"Teacher. What are you doing?"

The teacher calmly answered without turning his eyes from the two stones. "I am making a mirror."

"A mirror? Out of brick? But that's impossible. You are never going to be able to make a mirror out of brick."

Smiling, the teacher placed the bricks on the ground. "True son. This is very true. And in the same way; you will never ascertain grace or spiritual understanding by repeating two words over and over again." He then stood up and walked away, leaving the monk with his eyes wide open. [1]

This chapter is not designed to give you the step by step path of spiritual growth, but to call into question your feelings and understanding of the soul and the spirit. I want you to take a close look at what your current thoughts are about your spirit and ask yourself if you are simply rubbing two bricks together trying to make a mirror. Or, maybe you've reached the point where you've given up on even attaining a mirror at all so you believe that there is no use even trying. The honest realization of where you are is a great place to start this chapter.

What are you thoughts on the spirit?

Are you happy with where you are spiritually today? Why or why not?

_____
_____
_____
_____
_____
_____
_____
_____
_____
_____
_____
_____
_____
_____

It is important to start from the place where we understand where we are individually when it comes to the spirit because there is a specific call in our culture away from the spiritual side of life. In fact, there is a pulling away from all things spiritual. There is an overwhelming belief that if you can't see it, feel it, smell it or touch it, than it must not exist. It is an atheistic call away from all things spiritual and it is leaving many individuals in a conflicted place.

This is a very difficult truth for many of us to swallow, however, because we have an overwhelming sense in our hearts that there has to be more. There is a deeper understanding that this world is more than just stuff and that there is a greater purpose for our lives than simply getting the most money or learning the most facts and then leaving that knowledge or cash to the next generation. There is a rebellion in our hearts to this ideological concept.

Think about yourself. Have there been life moments that were supremely spiritual? Have there been times when you look back and say that there had to be more than just atoms and molecules guiding your steps? Have you sensed the call to a place of greater spiritual understanding? Because there truly is more to our life than just the flesh and bone of daily decisions mixed with the emotions of the past. There is a spiritual side to life.

"A life is either all spiritual or not spiritual at all. No man can serve two masters. Your life is shaped by the end your live for. You are made in the image of what you desire."

—**Thomas Merton** *(20th century Catholic monk, poet and social activist)*

Personally, I totally understand why many people in our culture have a hard time with the reality of spirit. Many times this difficulty comes from situations that they have been personally linked with or things that they have seen take place in the lives of those who were supposed to be highly "spiritual" or the manipulation of individuals who followed a certain spiritual path. I believe that this is why we have seen a dramatic shift away from a corporate form of spirituality to an individual form of spirituality in our culture. If it is all about ME, than I have a greater sense of control. If I am let down, then I have no one to blame but myself.

Even though there is great merit in an individual form of spirituality, there is a great strength when we link our personal spiritual lives with others who are seeking to live a life of the spirit. As we join arms, we can experience an exponential internal growth and allow that growth to greatly impact the lives of those that we have contact with each and every day. But, before we go there, let's look at what we are talking about when we make reference to the "spiritual" side of life.

The actual word **"spirit"** can be defined as **"breath"** and gives us the picture of a common story told from creation where God "breathed" into an inanimate Adam and life was created. This "breath" brought life. This "breath" brought spirit and actually became the driving force of humanity. And whether you are a creationist or an evolutionist, there has to be some validity behind a force that is within all living creatures that makes them different from those which are dead. Both the living and the dead have the same body parts and organs and molecular structure… but there is a force which brings life to the living. This force is spirit.

"We are not human beings on a spiritual journey. We are spiritual beings on a human journey."

—**Stephen Covey** *(20th century American author)*

Our beliefs and ideas of spirit really come to the forefront when we begin to tackle some of life's toughest questions. Take a moment and attempt to answer some of these questions:

THE BEST: A Life Manifesto

Who am I?

_____
_____
_____
_____
_____
_____
_____
_____
_____
_____

Why am I here?

_____
_____
_____
_____
_____
_____
_____
_____
_____
_____

Is this life and world any different because of my existence?

Am I more than what I look like or what I do?

For some of us, we have a firm understanding of our purpose and how the existence of spirit ties into this. For others, however, these are some of the toughest questions to answer and simply thinking about them calls us to deeper waters, drawing us into a spiritual journey that will last the rest of our lifetimes.

Whenever I talk about spirit to someone who is apprehensive or leery about what it actually means, I always share one of my favorite quotes when it comes to spirituality:

"Keep on asking, and you will receive what you ask for. Keep on seeking, and you will find. Keep on knocking, and the door will be opened to you." [1]

I am a firm believer that when you begin to walk in the direction of spirituality, those doors of your life will be opened and you will begin to move in a rhythm of understanding. Situation will lead to situation where your understanding will increase. You will begin to meet people who will cause you to have a greater understanding of spirit. You will come across books and teachings that will answer the questions that you are struggling with and seeking to understand. Truly, once you begin seeking, you are sure to find. Too many people in this life have just given up and concluded that they just weren't going to seek any more. For those individuals, they will never find because they are not looking.

As we do seek, however, we will find that the addition of new understanding will cause a greater awakening to take place in our lives. It is like a blindfold is being slowly lifted off of our eyes and we are able to see the world for the first time through the eyes of the spirit. Slowly, we begin to watch our lives move from spiritual death to life… from spiritual darkness to light.

So, the first step is a willingness to be open to the reality of spirit in our lives. Let's look at a couple things that we can do to practically embrace our spirituality.

Start Fresh Today: Even though this may be extremely difficult for some, I believe that it is vitally important. We need to move past those negative experiences that we had growing up or those terrible examples of spiritual leaders that we had in our lives and embrace the reality that everyone is not like that. Those who caused you pain or abuse were not good examples of what it means to live a spiritual life.

If you were abused sexually, physically, verbally or emotionally, the perpetrators were horrible spiritual examples to you. If you were made to feel like you were dirty or no good or nothing but a worthless sinner, they were abusing you and it was wrong. If guilt was a weapon used against you, this is simply a way that weak people seek to control and not a picture of true spirituality. Take a minute and write your past experience with spirituality and how that could shape your thoughts on it today.

_____
_____
_____
_____
_____
_____
_____
_____
_____

THE BEST: A Life Manifesto

_____
_____
_____
_____
_____
_____
_____
_____
_____
_____
_____
_____
_____
_____
_____
_____
_____
_____
_____
_____
_____
_____
_____
_____
_____
_____
_____
_____
_____

Now, I want you to do something that may be difficult, but is very necessary. I want you to grab some white out and paint over the words that you just wrote. Or, grab a thick black marker and put a line across it or highlight and delete your computer screen or simply take your pen and pencil and put X's all over the words that you just wrote. Because this is how things **were** and not how they **are**. Today, we begin anew.

Now, I want you to write what you believe healthy spirituality to be. Think about specific words that describe a healthy spirituality to you. Maybe you will use words like love, joy, peace, patience, kindness, goodness, gentleness, faithfulness or self control. Write some different words down that cause you to think about healthy spirituality and then explain what those descriptive words acted out would look like.

Actively Seek Out Spiritual Inlets or Outlets and Don't Be Afraid to Leave or Quit:

If you want to be actively seeking or walking down a spiritual path, then you need to be actively staying involved in the process. Your spiritual life is not a passive act, but an area where you need to stay actively involved. Your immediate response will be to return to those places or things that were your first influences to spirituality (e.g. the church of your youth, a spot in nature from childhood, etc.) and this is a very good first step. However, if these places caused you to distance yourself from spirituality in the past, you may have to allow yourself to leave or stop doing what you once did.

If you end up in a place that is just bringing back memories of shame and condemnation, you need to allow yourself the freedom to get as far away from that place as possible without feeling like you are running away from spirituality altogether. Personally, I am a Christian and Jesus Christ has done a magnificent work in my heart and life and I owe everything I have to Him, but there are churches all over this country that I would never want to go in to. They spew guilt and shame and condemnation and are far from the grace and full life that I experience through Jesus. Just because I am a Christian, doesn't mean that I have to openly embrace every other Christian organization in the world.

This is the same with you. If you find that something you are doing or a place that you are going is stirring up bad emotions from the past or pushing you away from your spirit, get up and go. Don't stop altogether, just stop what you were doing and start doing something else. Remember, this thing called life is a journey and you have to be willing to travel the road to get to where you want to be.

Seek out Others Who Are on the Path:

I am purposely very vague with this statement "on the path". Others don't necessarily have to be on *your* path, but they need to be on "the path". Find other people who are seeking to grow their spiritual muscles and become everything that they were created to be. Seek out and discuss your journey with others. In the same way that you need the wisdom and insight of others on your path, they also need your insight to continue down their path.

So many people believe that when they discover their path of spirituality that they are only to gather with like minded individuals. This belief has caused a huge segregation in the spiritual world that I believe has damaged and not strengthened it. If we are a Christian, why on earth are we afraid of being friends with a Buddhist? Or, if we are Muslim, why can't we befriend a Jew? There are often divisions even within a religion. Baptist Christians don't get along with Pentecostal Christians or Sunni and Shiite Muslims are consistently trying to murder one another. There needs to be an openness and love amongst people and if our spiritual path is really the true path, they will find it when they seek! But no one is ever going to understand if we are only singing "Kumbaya" in a corner with everyone who believes exactly how we do.

I believe that these steps will allow you to begin to rebuild your spiritual life and to have a positive impact on others, and ultimately the world. And isn't this really the main purpose of our lives? We all want to have a positive impact on this world and make it into a better place. And, sometimes that change is going to take place in our lives before it can ever be made anywhere else. We need to begin with that man in the mirror. And when we do, there are very visible and tangible benefits that take place. Here are a few:

Interconnectedness: When we are seeking to grow spiritually, there is a greater sense of oneness with the world and purpose in our hearts. We are no longer these directionless and chaotic piles of mass floating around in a universe. We have a purpose and that purpose is linked with the betterment of the world and humanity overall. We begin to see ourselves as a piece of the greatest puzzle of all time… mankind.

Purpose: I can think of nothing greater than the realization that I was created for a purpose. It is the same with you. Having a spiritual connectedness with the world allows you to have a greater understanding of the overall purpose of life. You have a mission or mandate to make this world into a better place. You have a responsibility to yourself and the overall planet to become the best person that you possibly can and accomplish more and more with each passing day.

"Efforts and courage are not enough without purpose and direction."

—John F. Kennedy *(35th President of the United States)*

Wisdom: There is a wisdom that comes from the spirit that far outweighs anything that can be linked with a book or simple higher education. Wisdom comes from within. Naguib Mahfouz, an Egyptian writer and Nobel winner said this: **"You can tell whether a man is clever by his answers. You can tell whether a man is wise by his questions."** Seeking spirituality in our lives causes us to continuously be questioning and poking and prodding. True spirituality causes us to increase in wisdom.

Creativity: There is an incredible spiritual side to creativity. If you ask any great artist or writer or actor, they will talk about a place that they tap in to in order to play the character or paint the masterpiece. Seeking spirituality in our lives will allow us to reach into an often untapped reservoir of creativity and ideas that has the power to greatly enhance our lives.

Freedom vs. Restriction: I often find people who tell me that they believe that spirituality is too restricting and will stop them from living the life that they want. I, however, have found just the opposite to be true. Spirituality is a truly freeing reality in my life. My spirituality has enabled me to learn and grow and follow the passions that dwell deeply in my heart. It has freed me and brought clarity to my mind and allowed me to bring inspiration into the world.

Ask yourselves some questions about what you just read:

Out of the three steps in Getting Started: "Start Fresh Today", "Spiritual Inlets and Outlets" and "Seeking Out Others", which one do I think I'm going to have the hardest time with and why?

_____
_____
_____
_____
_____
_____
_____
_____
_____
_____
_____
_____
_____
_____

What can I actively do to make this step easier in my life?

Out of the five benefits of spirituality, which one do I long for the most in my life and why?

What am I going to do this week to assure that I'm walking down the spiritual path and not simply standing at the trailhead watching everyone else go by?

_____
_____
_____
_____
_____
_____
_____
_____
_____
_____
_____
_____

I know that for some of us this journey is one that we have already started and we are enjoying every step of it. But I also know that there are some who are incredibly scared at what the future may hold. They have given up on spirituality long ago and are now contemplating the very first steps toward this great unknown. They feel like their legs aren't strong enough and that they may fall under the weight of their own bodies. This fear reminds me of a story:

There was a farmer who had acres of farmland that he would cultivate each year. One of his first years, he was plowing a certain area and he hit a spot that caused a loud noise and broke off one of the tines to his plow. He concluded that the area was filled with rocks and chose to simply avoid that area of land. In order to do this, he would pull off to one side as he neared the area and then bring the plow back on the path after a good quarter mile, leaving a large part of his field unplanted.

After about 15 years, the farmer was walking along in the field and tripped over something protruding from the ground. He looked down and it was a large boulder in the center of the unplanted stretch of field. He pulled the rock out and plunged his shovel into the fertile soil, realizing that it was soft and broke up easily. Moving to his feet he looked over the crops that were all around him and the empty stretch of land that he was standing on and shook his head. All these years this one rock had stopped a greater abundance in the life of this farmer's family. This one rock had stolen a great deal from this farmer. All the farmer had to do was deal with the rock.

Too many of us choose to simply "plow around" this subject of spirituality. We've been burned in the past and experienced difficulty because of it and we choose to say, "That ground's too rocky" and just plow around it. We miss a greater abundance in our lives because we choose to **avoid** instead of **address**. We need to get down on our knees and plunge our hands into the soil. We need to pull out that one boulder and feel the rich soil between our fingers. The soil that can bring life can also be the soil of our spirit.

Take that step today. Begin your spiritual journey and watch how you are transformed by your simple willingness to say, "I will seek…"

Epilogue: The End is Really the Beginning

Well, here we are at the end—or should I say the beginning? We have now reached the end of this book, but it will prove to become the very first chapter in the rest of our lives and this is the masterpiece that I'm really interested in reading.

> "What we call the beginning is often the end. And to make an end is to make a beginning. The end is where we start from."
>
> —T.S. Eliot *(20th century playwright and poet)*

I applaud you for putting in the work that you have... digging deep into your heart as you really work toward bringing yourself closer to THE BEST life ever. You now have a personal manifesto that will bring a revolution that will pour from your life into all that you come into contact with.

It starts today... in this moment... with this breath. This is the place where everything begins to change. You may have already started to see different areas of your life begin to change, but it is about to start moving at a faster rate as you live out the reality of the words that you have just read.

I want to encourage you and let you know that it can be done. Your life is not an accident and you have never been a mistake. There is a purpose and a destiny resting below the surface of your life just waiting to burst upon this world. And I believe that the time has now come for that explosion to take place.

Let me leave you with this final thought...

I read an article from the August 29, 1977 issue of Newsweek that talked about Elvis and a term that was made popular by his music—"All Shook Up". In fact, the article was entitled "All Shook Up" and talked about how Elvis was born an only child, dirt poor in a little town in Mississippi. He was a truck driver at the age of eighteen and decided one day to make a recording. The rest is history. Elvis became one of the most beloved musical artists of all time.

Just before his death, when Elvis was 42, he longed to just have a normal life and be able to walk on the sidewalk without being accosted for autographs or pictures. It is said that he would have paid a million dollars for simply one week of peace.

Pat Boone had said of him, "I cared a lot for Elvis. He went in the wrong direction. Ironically, we met for the last time when I was going toward the East and he was on his way to Las Vegas. He said to me, 'Say, Pat, where you going?' And I told him I was going to be involved in some kind of ministry. And he says, 'Hey, I'm going to Vegas. Pat, as long as I've known you, you've been going in the wrong direction.' Pat Boone answered, 'Elvis, that just depends on where you're coming from and where you're going.'"

In our lives, it is the same way. Are we going the right direction? Well, that depends on where we're coming from and where we are going. Choose wisely. Every breath is a gift from above.

Breathe deep.

Dream big.

Live life to the fullest…

Endnotes:

Chapter 2:

(1) Mother Teresa. "Mother Teresa: Come Be My Light– The Private Writings of the Saint of Calcutta". Doubleday, 2007. pp. 6-7.
(2) Covey, Stephen. "The Seven Habits of Highly Effective People". Simon and Shuster, 1989. p. 207.

Chapter 4:

(1) Lakein, Alan. "How to Get Control of Your Time and Your Life". Signet Publishing, 1973.
(2) Schimelpfening, Nancy. "Boundaries". 18 December 2007.
http://depression.about.com/od/glossary/g/boundaries.htm
(3) Cloud, Henry and John Townsend. "Boundaries: When to Say Yes, How to Say No to Take Control of Your Life." Zondervan, 1992.

Chapter 5:

(1) Collins, James and Jerry Porras. "Building Your Company's Vision." Harvard Business Review, Volume 74, Iss. 5. 1996. pp 65-77.

Chapter 6:

(1) Goetzke, Kathryn. "How Long Does it Take an Action to Become a Habit; 21, 28 or 66 Days?". 13 August 2011.
http://blogs.psychcentral.com/adhd/2010/05/how-long-does-it-take-an-action-to-become-a-habit-21-28-or-66-days

Chapter 7:

(1) The Web Team. "Expanding Your Amazing Neural Network". 2004. The Franklin Institute.
http://www.fi.edu/learn/brain/exercise.html#top
(2) The Web Team. "The Effects of Sleep Deprivation". 2004. The Franklin Institute.
http://www.fi.edu/learn/brain/sleep.html
(3) The Web Team. "A Healthy Diet May Be Important to Brain Health as Well as Body Health". 4 January 2011. National Institute on Aging.
http://www.nia.nih.gov/Alzheimers/Publications/ADProgress2005_2006/Part2/healthydiet.htm.htm

Chapter 8:

(1) Huesmann, L. Rowell and Jessica Moise-Titus and Cheryl-Lynn Podolski and Leonard D. Eron. "Longitudinal Relations Between Children's Exposure to TV Violence and Their Aggressive and Violent Behavior in Young Adulthood: 1977-1992". Developmental Psychology, Volume 39, No. 2.
(2) Marshall, W. L. "The Use of Sexually Explicit Stimuli by Rapists, Child Molesters, and Nonoffenders". The Journal of Sex Research 25, no.2. May 1988. pp. 267-88.

(3) Kaining, Kristin. "Does Game Violence Make Teens Aggressive?". 8 December 2006. MSNBC. http://www.msnbc.msn.com/id/16099971/ns/technology_and_science-games/t/does-game-violence-make-teens-aggressive/

(4) The Web Team. "Americans Watching More TV Than Ever; Web and Mobile Video Up Too". 20 May 2009. Nielson Wire. http://blog.nielsen.com/nielsenwire/online_mobile/americans-watching-more-tv-than-ever/

(5) The Web Team. "Effects of TV on the Brain". 2011. Erupting Mind. http://www.eruptingmind.com/effects-of-tv-on-brain/

Chapter 9:

(1) Nauert, Rick PhD. "Innately Drawn to Negative News". Online Posting. 28 August 2009. http://psychcentral.com/news/2009/08/28/innately-drawn-to-negative-news/8037.html

(2) National Highway Traffic Safety Administration. "National Statistics". Online Posting. 2010. Fatality Analysis Reporting System. http://www-fars.nhtsa.dot.gov/Main/index.aspx

(3) Holy Bible: New Living Translation. Proverb 16:28. Wheaton: Tyndale, 1996.

Chapter 10:

(1) Agin, Brent MD and Sharon Perkins RN. "What Happens to Aging Muscles". 2011. http://www.dummies.com/how-to/content/what-happens-to-aging-muscles.html

(2) Netter, Sarah. "Body Building Grandma Ernestine Shepherd Bench Presses, Runs Marathon at 73". 27

April. 2010. ABC News. http://abcnews.go.com/Health/mess-ernestine-shepherd-body-building-grandma-benches-150/story?id=10480184

(3) Inspired from: http://wserver.flc.losrios.edu/~willson/fitnessHandouts/muscleGroups.html

Chapter 12:

(1) Holy Bible: New Living Translation. Matthew 7:7. Wheaton: Tyndale, 1996.

ABOUT THE AUTHOR

GP Hintz is an author, speaker, and world traveler. From the slums of Brazil to the top of the Eiffel Tower, he journeys in order to hear the heart cry of humanity and capture it with words. He works tirelessly to help people grow in every area of their life, spiritually, mentally, physically and emotionally, and believes that everyone has profound purpose and a seed of destiny resting inside of them. He lives in Arizona with his wife and children.

Learn more about GP Hintz at his blog: gphintz.com or the book's website: thebestmanifesto.com.

www.ingramcontent.com/pod-product-compliance
Lightning Source LLC
Chambersburg PA
CBHW060823050426
42453CB00008B/561